ROARING BACK

ROARING BACK

THE FALL AND RISE OF TIGER WOODS

CURT SAMPSON

DIVERSION
BOOKS

For more information, email info@diversionbooks.com

Diversion Books
A division of Diversion Publishing Corp.
443 Park Avenue South, suite 1004
New York, NY 10016
www.diversionbooks.com

Book design by Neuwirth & Associates

First Diversion Books edition October 2019
Hardcover ISBN: 978-1-63576-683-7
eBook ISBN: 978-1-63576-682-0

Printed in The United States of America

1 3 5 7 9 10 8 6 4 2

Library of Congress cataloging-in-publication data is available on file.

In memory of Dan Jenkins.
His Ownself.

ROARING BACK

CONTENTS

Augusta Sky

The vintage single-engine Cessna traced lazy circles through the bright sunlight and broken clouds above Augusta. It was a gorgeous late spring day, the air having been washed clean by heavy rain after a long and uncharacteristic drought in east Georgia. The fifty shades of Augusta's April green had distilled down to eight or so; gone were chartreuse, lime, and tea, replaced by emerald, jade, sea, and dark.

"Dew point one seven six," droned the mechanical voice in my headset. "Visibility one zero miles." But I wanted to see farther than that. That was why we went up. With the 2019 Masters only six weeks in time's rearview mirror, I'd hoped an Olympian view would wake up the echoes and enable a more perfect recall of the drama that had occurred on the hilly acreage fifteen hundred feet below.

Pilot Mark Saisal flew our little red and white bird over the Savannah River, Interstate 20, several giant hospitals, neighborhoods both modest and grand, and the ragged shoreline of Lake Strom Thurmond in South Carolina. Then we looped back into the Peach State for more corkscrews over Augusta National and its next-door neighbor, Augusta Country Club. Printing executive and Augusta golf maven Tim Wright sat in the rear seat and pointed things out below us.

"Man, they're tearing up number thirteen," he said. A big swath of ground in front of the green on golf's greatest par four and a half was indeed denuded. "I wonder if they're putting in SubAir."

SubAir is an effective but very pricey underground vacuum system some usually very pricey clubs install under their greens, the better to keep the speed up and the ground dry even after it rains. I'd never heard of it being used beneath a fairway. "Can they do that?" I asked.

"Son, they can do whatever they want," Wright said. "Can you believe all the projects they got goin' on?"

I studied the ground, finding my way only very slowly, like a kid just learning to read. OK, there's number five, the hole they'd just lengthened into a killer of a par four. Boomerang-shaped thirteen was easy to recognize. There's the six and sixteen nexus. But where was the one hole, the *key* hole? Where's number twelve?

"There," said Wright. "See the black tarp in the bunker? They're keeping that white sand clean."

"Got it," I said, as I beheld the simplest-looking arrangement on the entire course: a blank little hill opposite a bean-shaped green, with a ribbon of shiny water unspooling between the two. But twelve had been like a dueling ground during the final few minutes of the 2019 Masters. Like the climax in the musical *Hamilton*, it was nine irons at one hundred and fifty paces. One man walked to the thirteenth tee unscathed while the others shot themselves in the feet, in a figurative sense.

As I stared down, I tried to picture the heroes and what they wore and the looks on their faces as they reacted to their fates. Woods, Finau, Koepka, and Molinari were compelling figures that day. Two of the wounded mounted brave comebacks, but the uninjured man proved to be braver still.

"Augusta tower this is Hotel seven seven niner requesting permission to land runway ten forty right over." Pilot Saisal is a big, bearded man who looks like he could rip the roof off a Range Rover, but he has a surgeon's touch with an airplane. Which is to say, the landing was as smooth as a baby's bottom.

"Thanks, Mark. Thanks, Tim," I said. The trip had given me the lay of the land better than I had ever had it; I saw, for example, how Rae's Creek feeds into the Savannah. On the other hand, the aerial view proved to feel a bit clinical and literally detached. We were too high to recreate the audience or the players in the recent drama.

All the emotion had been on the ground.

Green Beret's Boy

The father of the prodigy moved with ponderous dignity, like a yacht about to dock. On a sunny May day in 1993 in Irving, Texas, at TPC Las Colinas, during the first round of the GTE Byron Nelson Classic, sixty-one-year-old Earl Woods punched a walking stick into the ground with every second step. Below his beer barrel body, baggy Bermuda shorts revealed broomstick legs that looked inadequate for his weight or for the task at hand. He wore old man's white socks and sneakers, and mirrored aviator sunglasses. A pack of Merit 100 cigarettes fit snugly in his shirt pocket. The heart attack that loomed in '93 would strike three years later.

Inside the yellow nylon ropes, a much more vigorous specimen was busy shooting 77: Earl's whippet-thin seventeen-year-old son, Tiger, playing in his fourth PGA Tour event, and about to miss his fourth cut.

"Excuse me, Mr. Woods?" I said. Earl had paused for breath midway up the hill by the green on the seventh hole.

"I have two young sons at home, and I'm so impressed with the job you've done with Tiger . . ."

Earl knew what I wanted. By then he'd spoken with a hundred guys like me, probably a thousand. "First thing you do," he said, "Put a golf club in his crib."

We walked while he talked with the immobile face of a ventriloquist. While I'd expected a big dose of gung-ho from the former Green Beret, Lieutenant Colonel Woods presented a soothing voice, a quiet manner, and absolute confidence in the advice he was giving. The bogies being posted by his son seemed not to bother him in the slightest. What with the way we hung back from the action, and his eyes obscured by his shades, I couldn't tell if Papa Earl was even watching.

Meanwhile, in the arena on the other side of the ropes, Tiger frowned and ground away. His swing reminded me of the sudden blast of kinetic energy that might occur from the release of a big spring, an amusing metaphor I thought I might share if we met. Which we did, a couple of months later.

But before that, a word—a magic word—attached itself to Earl's fourth child. The word was *comeback*.

On July 31st, in the finals of the US Junior Amateur, at Waverley Golf Club, in Portland, Oregon, Tiger found himself two holes down with two to play. A win by the slim young man from suburban Los Angeles would be his third consecutive in the US Junior Am, a triple never before achieved (in fact, Jordan Spieth and Eun Jeong Seong, on the girls' side, are the only other multiple winners in the event's sixty-year history—both won twice).

"Tiger was clearly the best player in the field," recalls David Jacobsen, who with his younger brother, Peter, grew up playing Waverley.

"The sound of his club compressing the ball . . . wow. He hit lots of irons off the tee because he was so long."

Holding the lead and blocking Tiger's path to junior golf glory was another seventeen-year-old, Ryan Armour, a sturdy young man from Silver Lake, Ohio, which is near Akron. Ryan was bound for Ohio State; Tiger, Stanford. Armour needed only to tie the next hole or the one after that to win both the match and the tournament.

Bunkers left, the sun-dappled Willamette River right, and a big, excited gallery of five thousand all around. At the end point of the long uphill par four—Waverley's members played it as par five—lurked a narrow two-tiered green whose rear portion was as small as Melania Trump's walk-in closet and just as inaccessible: the seventeenth had been the toughest hole on the course all week. They'd cut the pin *just* on the edge of the top tier, and so far right it looked like it was off the green.

"Now let's see what Tiger's made of," Jacobsen said to a companion.

Adrenaline and the moment charged up both players. Armour hit three-wood, four-iron to the edge. Woods drew back on a driver—*sproing!* went the spring—and his ball rocketed into the middle of the fairway, far past his opponent's. Then he propelled his Titleist into the sky with a nine iron, landing it eight feet from the jar on the brick hard green, with so much spin that it stopped right there. The five thousand in attendance whooped it up. The Ohio boy chipped up close.

Silence. Tiger surveyed the grass between hole and ball as if searching for a contact lens. He murmured something to his caddie, a tall, low-key gentleman named Jay Brunza; usually it was clinical psychologist Brunza doing the soft talk. The former US Navy captain had been looping for and working with Earl's son since he was twelve and hypnotizing him since age thirteen.

"Immerse yourself mentally in the challenge of the moment," Brunza would say. "Remove the inhibition of fear. Harness self-belief and discipline."

Now Tiger lined up the putt and said: "Got to be like Nicklaus. Got to will this into the hole." With Jack-like will and a surgically precise tap with Tiger's Ping, the ball rolled in.

Woods managed to make himself a little miffed when he saw that Armour was playing for a par five on Waverley's 578-yard eighteenth. *He doesn't think I can make a birdie! I'll show him!* And he did, with the last two shots being a forty-yard bunker shot to another hidden pin and a ten-foot putt. Tiger won the thing with a par on the first extra hole. That's what Tiger was made of, Mr. Jacobsen. What a comeback!

"It was mine, I had it in my hands, but he was teasing

me," Armour said afterwards. "It was like he was following a script."

Fate decreed that David J. would get another emphatic illustration of young Tiger's genius the next summer, when the two stud golfers—one age 42, the other 18—met in the semi-finals of the Pacific Northwest Amateur, at Royal Oaks Country Club in Vancouver, Washington.

Jacobsen, who was only marginally less good a golfer than his famous younger brother, held the phenom to a tie after nine holes. With the honor, the older man drove straight and long on the par four tenth; Woods snap-hooked a two iron into the woods. Tiger chipped out. David hit an iron to within a step or two of the pin. Tiger holed his shot from 100 yards. David, shaken and stirred, missed his short putt and lost the hole.

About a minute later in golf time, the teenager produced birdie-birdie-birdie-eagle-handshake. The gracious loser approached the father of the winner to say something nice. And Earl said, without irony, "That took longer than I thought it would." Bam. And ouch.

The USGA's next big event after the Junior at Waverley was the US Amateur, which was held at Champions Golf Club in Houston. Back then I was writing for *Golf Journal*, the USGA's magazine. Editor David Earl suggested I get an eyeful of and then an earful from the wondrous young man who'd just won his third consecutive Junior. Will do, I said, but I didn't. Not the second part, anyway.

Galleries were slim to non-existent for first round matches in the debilitating Houston heat and humidity—Earl did not walk through that outdoor sauna, thank goodness—but it was no hardship for me to watch straw-hatted Tiger, a skinny little maestro in an enormous golf shirt. Besides, he ended his match with dispatch. After he shook his opponent's hand on the fourteenth green, I approached, explained my mission, and offered my own hand. Or, from his point of view, a dead fish wrapped in newspaper.

Tiger's limp grip hinted at his lack of interest. Nor would he make eye contact, instead finding something more interesting to look at in the distance over my left shoulder. Ignoring the plain-as-day body language, I said, "May I ask you a couple of questions now? Or, if you prefer, back at the clubhouse? I wouldn't mind some air-conditioning!"

"Maybe later," he said, plainly meaning "probably never," and walked away. I was left open-mouthed at so thorough a brush-off.

Tiger lost the next day, two and one, to Englishman Paul Page. A forty-one-year-old Minnesotan named John Harris won the event. The USGA's photographer mentioned that he'd done all his complicated set-up for a scheduled photograph of the Junior champ, but the champ did not show. "He's sure to be a superstar. He's already acting like one," the shooter said.

My review in the magazine included a slightly snippy sentence about Tiger. Which was petty. And uninformed: who knew the bickering between his parents was making Tiger's home life a depressing mess? I didn't. A more sympathetic reporter might also have taken a long look at the emotional cost of being a celebrity all his life. Had Eldrick T. been rude to me or just very wary? Both, I think.

But forget the '93 US Amateur, unless to raise a glass to Harris. Instead let's remember what happened a year later, in the same event, when that magic word reattached to Tiger. In the US Am's 36-hole final at TPC Sawgrass, Woods was getting walloped by a wonderful young player from North Texas named Trip Kuehne, pronounced key-knee, brother of Hank, the US Amateur champ of 1998 and Kelli, who won the US Girls Junior and the Women's Am twice. Kuehne led by six holes with thirteen holes to play—a foreshadowing phrase if ever there was one—but then Tiger did what he did, did what he again does. He made long putts, chipped in for par with the pin out, played a couple of great shots from the woods, bounced one off a pine tree on sixteen, "was lucky as hell" on seventeen, as he admitted, and finished birdie-birdie-par on TPC's fierce final three.

"The Comeback Kid: Tiger Woods Wins '94 US Am" was the USGA's headline, and the one used by *Sports Illustrated*. He won the next Am, too, at Newport Country Club, over a man old enough to be his father, and the one after that at Pumpkin Ridge, Portland, in a comeback that echoed his junior triumph at Waverley, for three Ams in a row. No one had ever done that before, not even the greatest-ever amateur,

Bobby Jones. Woods turned pro in the fall of '96 amid unprecedented hoopla and hype. Nike and Titleist paid him a combined $60 million and both got their money's worth. His win in the '97 Masters knocked the world for a loop. He kept winning.

Now, after setbacks that would have floored a lesser performer, and after what happened in April in Augusta, the Comeback Kid is now the Comeback Man.

But there are comebacks and there are Comebacks. Within the lowercase version are quick-witted quips, as from a comedian to a heckler ("why don't you go stand in the corner and finish evolving") or between debating politicians ("Senator, you're no Jack Kennedy") and the rich tapestry of putdowns and zingers from wits such as Dorothy Parker ("if you want to know what God thinks of money, just look at the people he gave it to"), Alice Roosevelt Longworth ("If you don't have anything nice to say, come sit by me"), Winston Churchill ("Ramsay MacDonald is a sheep in sheep's clothing"), and David Feherty ("that ball is so far left Lassie couldn't find it if it were wrapped in bacon").

There are also all manner of professional, personal, and political comebacks and—the point here—athletic ones. But in no game, including the game of life, is overcoming more important and more constant than in golf. Because virtually every imperfect shot requires the golfer to recover to some degree and almost all shots are imperfect. Those of us who give up a little after a bad bounce or a buried bunker ball watch the game on TV or from the civilian side of the gallery ropes. The talented few who can deal with adversity are the ones who play in the big leagues.

Resilience even has a metric. While stats-mad baseball may have an HRASO category for the plucky sluggers who hit a homerun in their next at-bat after striking out, professional golf has Bounce Back, and it's a Thing as much as Greens in Regulation or Sand Saves are. Bounce Back is the percentage of times a player makes a birdie after a bogey. The best—Brooks Koepka and Francesco Molinari, for instance, are in the top ten as of this writing—bounce back about a third of the time. The mighty Koepka fell very low then bounced very high when he followed a double bogey with an eagle on holes twelve and thirteen in the final round of the 2019 Masters. If not for that water ball on twelve . . .

A small number of golf comebacks deserve a capital C and make us stop and think about mountains climbed and the weight on the climber's back. For example: not many climbed as high and with a greater load than the first great black player on the PGA Tour. No, not grouchy Charlie Sifford or placid Lee Elder, both of whom were good but far from great, and not Tiger. This man's name was Calvin Peete and he was born four down.

Calvin grew up poor in a crowded house in Detroit, the eighth (or ninth; accounts vary) child of Irenna and Dennis Peete, an auto worker. Dennis added ten more kids to the clan with his second wife. It's sad but no surprise that with so many feet to shod and noses to wipe, Calvin was farmed out to his grandma. She lived in Hayti—pronounced hay-tie—a garden spot on the Mississippi River in southern Missouri.

Grandma had a cherry tree. One day twelve-year-old Calvin climbed it, then fell out of it, breaking some combination of humerus, radius, and ulna in his left elbow. It may be a commentary on the quality of orthopedic surgery in Greater Hayti that Calvin could never straighten that arm again, not even close.

Next came a migration to another agricultural outpost—Pahokee, on Lake Okeechobee in central Florida, because Calvin's father had moved there. Pahokee and neighboring Belle Glade—aka "Muck City"—promised hot weather, rich land for sugar cane, fruit, and vegetables, and hard work and poverty for ten-dollar-a-day bean and corn pickers like young Calvin. Away from the field, the thin young man learned the basics of cigarettes, dice, pool, and cards, and made room for them by dropping out of school for good after the eighth grade.

When Calvin looked past the next row of bean poles, he beheld a grim future, but then came an idea, and a turning point: Grandma financed the purchase of an old car that the new entrepreneur filled with stuff to sell to the people he knew best, migrant farm workers. He migrated slowly north with them as the seasons and the crops changed. It was citrus, lettuce, beans, corn, blueberries, plums . . . Calvin's mobile store was a good idea because the bosses gave the pickers so little time to shop. *"Miro esto,"* the salesman would say, leading the *recolectors de fruta* to his tail-finned '56 Plymouth Suburban station wagon. Look at this dress, shirt, blanket, blender, knick-knack, whatever. To goose sales in the jewelry division of Calvin Peete Inc., he made himself a walking advertisement: any time he smiled, you saw the diamonds he had embedded in his two front teeth.

Let's skip ahead to the fall of 1966, harvest time in Upstate New York. The Diamond Man, now age twenty-three, is in Rochester to work the apple pickers' camps. Some friends—part-time caddies at Genesee Valley Golf Course—inveigle him to try golf for the first time. He resists. But rather than wait in the car, he tries it. He swings and misses or hits grounders all day. Stupid game. What does a poor black man with a crooked arm want with golf? What does golf want with him?

For the answer to that question, let's time travel again, to the early morning of March 31, 1985. The former Diamond Man—he's had his dental gems removed—is so nervous he can't sleep. He creeps out of bed in the middle of the night, gets behind the wheel of a borrowed car, and drives for a few aimless hours up and down A1A in north Florida. At one point he turns on the interior light and inclines the rearview mirror so he can look himself right in the eye. "You know what, Calvin?" he says. "You have an opportunity . . . When you at your best they can't beat you. They can't beat you."

And they couldn't. A final round 66 gave the quiet man

in a Kangol hat a win by three in the Players Championship, which some allege is golf's fifth major. The former bean picker who never had a lesson or much support from anybody ended his career with fourteen professional wins—twelve in the US, two in Japan—and ten years in a row as the tour's straightest driver. He got his GED because the PGA required its Ryder Cup players to have a high school diploma. He played in two Ryder Cups, won a Vardon Trophy for the tour's lowest stroke average, and had eight children, among them Calvin and Kalvanetta.

There's another number to think about: the number of times the only black player in the field was asked in a clubhouse "who are you caddying for?" He didn't count. It happened a lot.

Peete died at age 71, in Atlanta, of lung and pancreatic cancer. "A tremendously warm and caring man," eulogized his contemporary and peer, Jack Nicklaus. "He gave so much of himself to the game and to others."

Clearly, Calvin Peete's comeback from the circumstances life threw at him had a different flavor than Tiger's inspirational triumph in the 2019 Masters. No one ever held Calvin out as a savior or as the avatar of a new era of racial harmony. The humble former farm worker and traveling salesman made only a modest splash in America's popularity pool even with his big win in the '85 Players. Tiger's impact, on the other hand, was that of a fat kid executing a cannonball.

Calvin had a bent wing, but Tiger's jacked-up back had

him crawling as much as walking two years before the events in April 2019 in Augusta. Peete suffered from wheezy lungs and from Tourette syndrome, an annoying neurological disease that caused him to twist and turn his head and neck and which was not diagnosed until his career was virtually over. But Tiger was in so much physical and psychic pain two years ago that his very survival was in question. That's not an exaggeration: just look at his tox screen after his traffic arrest at 2 a.m. on that Monday morning in May 2017.

So now we contemplate the hero to zero back to hero journey of Eldrick Tont "Tiger" Woods. His story seems to have no peer or precedent, but it can be illuminating to compare things to the incomparable.

How do other presidents stack up against Abraham Lincoln? The answer reveals a lot about Lincoln.

PART ONE

The Hogan Thing

"Much wants more."

—Jack Burke, Jr., 1956 Masters and PGA champion

The fall and rise of Tiger Woods is marked by so many distinct milestones that to calculate the distance between zenith and nadir we have to take the full measure of Tiger's leap toward immortality at the 1997 Masters. So, before we look at his win in 2019, let's reconsider his triumph in the first one, twenty-two eternal summers previously. That April 7 through 13 in Augusta, Georgia felt so ratcheted-up and fraught that it seemed oddly unreal. Tournament badges were going for $8,000 and up, for God's sake. Because of Tiger. Because he was going to win.

Twenty-something years is long enough ago for things to have been a little different. On the course, the squared-off, ten-gallon golf hat was a look, and driver club heads were metal, but they were small, about half the size of today's canned hams. The Chicago Bulls outlasted the Utah Jazz in the NBA Finals, the Florida Marlins prevailed in seven games over the Cleveland Indians in the World Series, and the Denver Broncos won the Super Bowl, beating the Green Bay Packers, in January. *Titanic* was the movie, "Don't Talk" the song, and Miss America hailed from Kansas. Princess Diana died, as did Mother Theresa.

And Augusta was delirious, and not because a local woman, Lt. Commander Susan Still, had piloted the space shuttle as it took off a week before the Masters. I bumped around town as if in a dream along with everyone else. Compared to all prior years, according to the experts I was about to meet, the traffic was more snarled, the scalpers and scalpees more numerous and high-strung, and the pools around town splashed with unprecedented cash. Pools meaning betting pools; if you're invited to an Augusta pool party, bring your wallet, not a swimsuit.

Two days before the tune-a-mint, while seated at the crazily crowded counter to the left of the cash register at the Waffle House by the Bobby Jones Expressway, an arm appeared in the middle of my sports page, as if by magic. "Danny Fitzgerald"—accent on the Fitz—said the bald man attached to the arm. "How you doin'? Where you from?"

Not two minutes later, Arnold Palmer, party of four, walked into the Waffle House by the Bobby Jones Expressway. More magic as the money spot—the booth at the restroom end—suddenly became available. The people applauded and shouted "Arnie!" The handsome king in a cardigan beamed, waved, ordered eggs. Everyone in the jam-packed space seemed over-the-moon happy, Christmas Eve happy. Because

Arnie was in the house. And because of Tiger, who was going to win.

I was in attendance to bear witness and to otherwise continue research on a book about the club, the town, and the tournament (daringly entitled *The Masters*) and I wanted to meet people. Boy, did I meet people. With the ebullient Fitz as my guide and translator, it was "this is Mayor Sconyers of the great city of Augusta, Georgia" and say hi to this Augusta National member or this other one and let's go have a chat with Byron Nelson. Through friendly natives Danny and Tim Wright and their cadre of friends, I learned the True Meaning of the Masters, which is that it's a ritual, and a reunion, with white water rafting on a river of beer. I needed a life jacket. For local aficionados in particular, the Masters is golf Mardi Gras. It's got everything but a parade and show us your beads.

But on the cold Saturday morning of that giddy week, I was shocked to be attending a funeral for a friend of a new Augusta friend. Allen F. Caldwell III had shot and killed himself the day before. He'd been a ticket broker. Skyrocketing demand from corporate customers and broken promises had ruined him financially in the blink of an eye. That sad footnote dampened the joy of the week for relatively few people and that's a good thing, but I dwelled on it.

We certainly can't lay this at Tiger's feet. Can't blame him for being too charismatic and this opportunity too historic. And not that they had any responsibility for Mr. Caldwell, either, but we can mention two entities that stirred the pot. Who to fire at first? Nike, your honor.

Talking here about the marketing giant's unctuous, pandering, and extremely effective commercial that had been released to coincide with Tiger's professional debut seven months earlier, in September '96. Against purposely blurred or grainy images of Tiger making putts and throwing celebratory fists, "Hello, World" was a sort of call and response, but with no voice-over, just a drumbeat and an echoing choir, and words on the screen that said, in part:

I won the US Junior when I was 15.
Hello, world.
I played in the Nissan Open when I was 16.
Hello, world . . .
I am the only man to win three consecutive US Amateur titles.
Hello, world.
There are still courses in the US I am not allowed to play because of the color of my skin.
Hello . . .

What in the world? Notwithstanding the fact that the world and Tiger were obviously already well-acquainted, playing the race card in this first big commercial message seemed especially tasteless. It wasn't a worthy way to sell shirts and shoes. And the very idea that any course in the world would not unroll its reddest carpet for the blossoming global superstar was ludicrous.

Besides, Ambassador of his Race was a job Tiger seemed reluctant to embrace, and who could blame him? The only time he even thought about ethnicity, he said, was when writers asked him about it, and he was emphatic that he did not wish to be referred to as black. Race isn't only about melanin, of course: Tiger lived in a white town (according to the 2000 census, of the 46,229 people in Cypress, CA, 2.7 percent were black), played a white sport at a white high school, and his friends and girlfriends were white. He wasn't black in the way that most white Americans think of being black. Fed up with all the really-none-of-your-business questions, recall Tiger's presentation of a portmanteau word to describe his racial makeup; he was Cablanasian, he explained, not Caucasian, black, or Asian. He was all three.

Writers called them out—the global marketing giant and its ad agency. Well, we didn't mean it *literally*, they admitted. It's a metaphor. Hmmm. Nike seemed to be hiding behind the concept of puffery, the legal term for promotional statements that may not be objectively true. Lucky Charms are not really magically delicious, for example, and the low, low prices at Crazy Dan's Discount Mattress Warehouse are not actually insane. But "I'm not allowed to play because of the color of my skin" wasn't playful or funny, nor was it transparent. It was simply dishonest.

That spot had legs, however, and defenders, and people

remembered it long after it had been replaced by the next one, in which kids of all races and both genders declare "I Am Tiger Woods." They weren't. It was a metaphor. This qualifies as actual puffery, we suppose, but again with the race-based selling strategy. They could have gone in so many other directions.

Earl roiled the waters as much as Nike did and more often. The grandiosity of his statements astonishes even now. According to *Tiger Woods,* the estimable 2018 biography by Jeff Benedict and Armen Keteyian, the son cringed when his father said the heretofore unsayable, even by Mohammed's pop, and Joseph of Nazareth, and Charlie Nicklaus.

Earl's motivation couldn't be clearer: he was aggrieved from his treatment by the majority race throughout his life, including, surprisingly, his twenty years in our purest melting pot, the US military. Earl seemed to want to get even through his son. During Tiger's first presser as a golf professional, pops averred that Tiger "would do more than anyone in human history to change the course of humanity," more, even, than Buddha, Gandhi, or Nelson Mandela. Please.

Earl addressing the press wasn't part of Team Tiger's choreography that day, but he plainly wanted his share of the spotlight and thought he deserved it. How else are we to explain him?

At a college golf awards banquet, in his introduction to the main honoree (guess who), Earl shared "that I know I was personally selected by God himself to nurture this young man." What a thought, and what a choice of words. *Personally* selected. God could have asked his secretary to handle it, but no.

In the afterglow of Tiger's second consecutive US Amateur win at swanky Newport (Rhode Island) Country Club, Earl did some standup but got no laughs. He'd had a few. He held a drink in one hand and the Havemeyer trophy in the other.

"How do you like this, Bobby Jones?" asked the proud, embarrassing papa. Someone should have hit a snare drum.

"A black man is the best golfer who ever lived."

"Bobby Jones can kiss my son's black ass."

Cablanasian ass, Earl.

Jones, the cofounder of Augusta National and of the Masters, and one of the game's enduring heroes, had been dead since 1971 and could neither take offense nor smooch. With time and success and very respectful treatment by the people who ran the event, Earl came to love the place as others did. "It's like God designed this as a golf course," he told *Golf Digest* in 2008. "It's a shrine, really."

But back then, Earl and Tiger had Charlie Sifford in their ears. They loved the guy. Charlie hated the Masters.

Mr. Woods and Mr. Sifford bonded over the slights and racial injustice they'd both suffered as young men. Earl had been a pretty good baseball player in Kansas back in the day. He was a catcher—the position reserved for the best athlete, he said—and was the only person of color on his youth all-star team, at the state youth tournament, at Kansas State, and in the entire Big 8 Conference. You know this story: hotels refused to let him check in. Restaurants wouldn't serve him even though he was with the team. *Inferior* white people would not treat him as an equal.

Ditto Charlie, in golf. The ex-caddie from Charlotte turned pro at age seventeen and won the Negro National Open six times. But he couldn't prove himself—or make a decent income—by succeeding in the tournaments you read about in the paper. Why not? Three letters: PGA.

Although the Professional Golf Association of America had not allowed blacks or women since its inception in 1916, in 1934 they'd codified their racial discrimination by inserting Article III, Section 1 into their by-laws: the infamous "Caucasians only" clause. History is looking at you, presidents of the PGA of America during the twenty-seven years the whites-only rule was in effect. Two in particular were notable in that they looped back to Augusta: Ed Dudley held the PGA helm from 1942 to 1948. Big Ed, who won fifteen times on the tour, was also the pro at Augusta National since its founding in '32 and for twenty-five years thereafter.

Another interesting prez in this era was Horton Smith, who led the PGA from '52 to '54. Yes, that Horton Smith, the Horton Smith who won the first Masters in 1934 and the third one two years later. The wavy-haired, no-smoke, no-drink man from Missouri had two other substantial attachments to Augusta: he married a local gal, an heiress named Barbara Bourne, the daughter of an original member of Augusta National; and he had a long, friendly association with club and tournament co-founder Bobby Jones, whose affectionate nickname for him was The Tall Boy. Horton had been one of Bobby's main rivals in his Grand Slam year of 1930. With the 1954 Supreme Court decision in *Brown v. Board of Education* outlawing segregated schools, and many other efforts to mitigate American apartheid, the issue of admitting black members was in the wind more than ever during Smith's PGA presidency. Professional baseball, basketball, and football had all already integrated, and hockey would follow soon after.

Golf's Negro league—the United Golfers Association—produced some pretty good players after World War II besides Sifford, among them Teddy Rhodes and Bill Spiller. When Rhodes and Spiller seemed to have qualified for a PGA tournament but then were not allowed to tee it up, they boiled over. How can you keep anyone out of a tournament with a qualifying system and called an "open"? Rhodes and Spiller hired a lawyer, who prepared a lawsuit against the PGA demanding $250,000 in damages. President Smith promised to right this wrong if the suit was dropped—it was—but instead of reform, the PGA dragged its bureaucratic feet and then merely changed one word. Henceforth its tournaments would not be called Opens; they'd be Invitationals or "Open Invitationals," a contradictory term if ever there was one. Negroes were simply not invited. See? No discrimination.

Sifford, who was ten years older than Earl, had a swing

like a punch to the gut, a double Corona clamped in the corner of his yap, and an attitude. During his wasted prime, all he got from dominating the UGA tour was small checks and big frustration. After twenty years in the wilderness, the PGA—under legal pressure—finally let him play in 1961. Professional golf was behind the times; the Boston Red Sox, the last major league team to integrate, had done so one year earlier. Sifford went through hell that first year. In Greensboro, he received death threats that seemed quite credible, and an extremely unpleasant gang of white boys coalesced in his gallery and shouted the things racist dumbasses shout. Charlie was supposed to be eligible for the tournaments in Houston and San Antonio but when he drove up, he was turned away. Better late than never, the PGA erased the Caucasian clause from the books at its annual meeting that November.

Cigar-chomping Charlie made up for lost time to a degree, but he was bitter and grew even more so when he won a couple of regular tour events but was not invited to play in the Masters. "Them motherfuckers kept me out," he told me in 1996. *"Fuck* Cliff Roberts"—Roberts being Jones's partner and co-founder of Augusta National and the Masters and also quite dead. The situation was more complicated than Charlie and his supporters portrayed, however. Over the years several white players who'd won a tour event also did not get a parking spot or a locker at Augusta National in April. But Sifford went through a lot and he told Tiger about it.

Which brings us back to east Georgia in 1997 and the gathering of pilgrims expecting to witness the Tiger miracle, with many, many millions more focused on the flickering screens in their homes and in 19th holes around the country. How many millions more? About forty-four for Sunday, which was a record. Which was crazy, because there would be no real competition that day. I guess we all just wanted to see the coronation. After three rounds, Tiger led by *nine* over Signor Costantino Rocca of Ferragamo, Italy, who was a good player who had nearly won the previous Open Championship but was no one to fear. He had a smile on his face and CLUB MED on his hat.

"There's a new era about to dawn at the most magical setting in golf," said announcer Jim Nantz as the show opened. "A place where legends are made. Where dreams have been realized. Where the royalty of the game have driven down Magnolia Lane to find their golf kingdom . . ."

Way back on Thursday, the new royal had shot a fat four-over forty on the front nine. But then a comeback ensued, a big one. For the next sixty-three holes—for the remainder of the tournament, that is—Tiger shot twenty-two under par. *That* was crazy! His win set all sorts of records, including biggest-ever margin of victory in the Masters, twelve—as you probably already know.

"Can't believe he's only twenty-one," announcer Ken Venturi said. About ten times.

With the final putt holed, the crowd roared, and the

young man in red and black hugged his caddie, Michael "Fluff" Cowan—who was on permanent loan from Peter Jacobsen—for two seconds. Tida, his mother, also got two. In between them, Earl, who was barely ambulatory six weeks after triple bypass surgery, embraced his son for twenty-two camera-hogging seconds. Time would reveal the dark corners of Tiger's paternal inheritance; eventually, the son would have to overcome his father, as most sons must in one way or another. But in this moment, their debt to each other and their love for each other could not be missed.

The new champ was poised during the Presentation of the Threads in the Butler Cabin. Before not-yet-Sir Nick Faldo helped him into a 42L and said something about the new champ's red top clashing with his green jacket, Nantz posed an extraordinary two-part question. Paraphrasing here—Nantz asked: as the first African-American *and* the first Asian-American to win the Masters—how does it feel?

Wow—a lot of taters in that sack, Jim. But Tiger nailed it.

"I may be the first, but I wasn't the pioneer," Tiger said. And he invoked the names of Sifford, Spiller, and Rhodes.

• • •

The time I didn't really meet him at the '93 US Amateur in Houston, Tiger made a far, far more important acquaintance. One day that week, he drove west and south from Champions to a pampered acreage near George Bush Intercontinental Airport. He told the guard his name and then was admitted to Houston's luxurious same-sex golf club.

"Hi, Butch."

"Nice to meet you, Tiger."

For the virtuoso performers and high-maintenance perfectionists at the top of professional golf and tennis, a coaching change is a very big deal. John Anselmo, Tiger's coach for the previous seven super-successful years, was out. The kindly Huntington Beach-based pro had been handy geographically—his course, Meadowlark Golf Club, was just a thirty-minute drive from the Woods house in Cypress. But now Anselmo was ageing, ill and out of action due to colon cancer. Besides, Earl desired a teacher with a bigger reputation and with more experience working with tour players. Greg Norman ranked number one or two in the world back then. His guy would do.

Claude Harmon, Jr.—aka "Butch"—was the oldest son of the 1948 Masters champion and brother to three other highly-thought-of instructors. He hung out a shingle at Lochinvar, an oil zillionaire's club that took its men-only policy very seriously. That a woman from the United States Postal Service breached the gate every day to deliver the checks and bills so annoyed the club that, according to legend, it moved its mailbox out to the street.

Eldrick and Claude clicked immediately. The new instructor agreed to start a tab; the Woodses had no money to pay him just then, but they would in time. Now military men filled all three spots on the teenager's advisory board. Earl, of course; caddie/sports psychologist Brunza; and the rough, tough, hard-to-bluff former infantryman. Harmon led a mortar team in 'Nam and doesn't want to talk about it, but he'll never forget it. Photos on the website for his golf school show Butch in camo, worn to illustrate his support for fellow vets.

In addition to a deep understanding of theory, practice, and blunt but effective communication skills, Harmon had another attractive attribute: a strong connection to Golf Jesus.

I'm talking about the patron saint of the practice tee, the game's research scientist, the author of its textbook, and one of its greatest players: William Ben Hogan.

Hogan was a shy man isolated by his obsessions and by the fact that, unlike almost everyone else, he traveled the tour with his wife. The Hawk didn't have or need a lot of friends, but he liked Butch's dad, also Claude Harmon, the pro at Winged Foot Country Club. The pals were paired in the '47 Masters. Harmon aced the twelfth hole.

"I had two, Claude," said Hogan on the walk to the thirteenth tee. "What did you have?" Or, in another version of the oft-told story, Hogan said nothing at all, so wrapped up in himself and his game that he noticed nothing else.

The next April, on the trek back north from his winter job at Seminole, in south Florida, Claude paused to win the Masters of 1948, by five, a record. Then the family rolled on home to New York.

The Harmons' backyard could be an exciting place during those summers. While steaks cooked on the grill and six kids scooted around, an honored guest would swirl the ice in his glass. "Show me your swing," Ben Hogan would say to the Harmon boys.

"Dad could get him to relax, to have a few Scotches," Butch told me in '95. "[Hogan] was a little insecure, had a little inferiority complex. That's why he was perceived as arrogant. Back then I noticed how he went for ultimate perfection when he mixed the drinks."

Claude revered the man. So did his oldest boy. On the day the three teed it up together, the youngster was just too nervous to function. "About the third hole," Butch recalled in a 2016 interview with the Westchester *Journal News,* Uncle Ben told him to just relax—it's only golf. "And I'm like, 'are you kidding me?' I'm playing with God!"

In the wake of his game-changing win in the '97 Masters, and again, in 2019, aficionados searched for someone worthy of comparison to Tiger. And the name that kept coming up was God—that is, Hogan. Their similarities lay in their dedication to practice; the explosive strength of their swings— while also somehow remaining perfectly balanced; their willingness to work the ball high or low, or left to right or right to left as the occasion demanded, no matter the pressure of the moment. The sheer athleticism in their skinny bodies. Their relentlessness. Their aloofness.

One cool, sunny day in the early aughts, Tiger channeled

Ben quite succinctly, by going out to the great man's club and hitting his clubs.

Nike's golf club testing and development center was in Fort Worth, Hogan's hometown, not far from Shady Oaks Country Club, where the ageing champion spent many happy hours with the love of his life: practice. Often it was practice with a purpose, for Hogan had his own equipment company, and he was the prototype tester. Upon his arrival, Tiger met with Shady Oaks head pro Mike Wright to select some Hogan-played Hogan clubs to hit. "Tiger had the most amazing personal presence," Wright recalls. "In my life, I've only seen that level of charisma in one other person—Mr. Hogan."

Wright led Tiger and his team of ten out to Shady's par-three course—what they call the Little Nine—and pointed out the secluded patch of ground Hogan used as his launching pad.

A camera crew shot from different angles and Nike executives Kel Devlin and Tom Stites looked on while Tiger, in conservative colors and baggy, pleated pants that Hogan would have approved of, swung away for a long time. What impresses most from the video Wright shot that day was how quickly Tiger was able to move those leaden cudgels through the air. Every component of the forty-year-old sticks—grip, shaft, and head—weighed way more than what's in use today, and they were balanced differently. Yet Tiger slashed with his usual controlled violence and with what looked like the same speed.

"Until Tiger came along," Butch said, "I'd never seen a good player with body speed as fast as Mr. Hogan's."

Mister Hogan. No one says Mr. Nicklaus or Mr. Palmer or Mr. Woods and Nelson would say, "call me Byron" as soon as he got to know you. But those in the loop always use the honorific. Hogan liked the distance contained in the formal title, and he was not just another Ben.

Although that's how Tiger refers to him; he's on a first name basis with his late peer.

Mister Hogan had been top of mind for golf instructors since the 1957 publication of *Five Lessons: The Modern Fundamentals of Golf,* by Himself with an assist from Herbert Warren Wind. For good and ill—it taught a world of slicers how to *never* hit a hook and it got teachers teaching the game all wrong, like a geometry lesson—it is easily the best-selling golf instruction book of all time. It continues to sell to this day. When there's a pause in the conversation, or he's trying to get you to stop re-gripping at the top, notice how often your pro will begin a sentence with "Mr. Hogan always said . . ."

But except for his gaudy golf record, no one really knew too much about the man, who was private, almost reclusive. I wrote his bio and called it *Hogan*, a simple title for a complicated man. "Boy, when I started reading it, I couldn't put it down," the highly unlikely 1996 US Open champion told the press late on a June Sunday afternoon at Oakland Hills Country Club. Steve Jones had just won by one over Tom Lehman. "And honestly I don't think I could have won this tournament without reading that book. Sounds crazy . . ."

Jones said *Hogan* gave him a new appreciation for how fiercely the man focused. Other readers enjoyed having Ben's most basic facts filled in, such as his full name, where he was born, and whether he really was left-handed. Others liked the book because they didn't know about the Comeback or wanted to be reminded of it.

Hogan's against-the-odds revival took place seventy years before Tiger roared back in Augusta. Now everyone's comparing them again.

Hogan's nightmare began when four three-hundred-pound linemen whose mothers never hugged them took a running start and slammed into him with all they had. Or, that was what it was like, approximately, when the 346 cubic inch Cadillac monoblock flathead V-8 engine shot like a made-in-Detroit missile through the firewall of the car and into the body of the seated, defenseless man. Many bones broke simultaneously—pelvis, ribs, shoulder, ankle—but a hard shot to the left side of the head, which punched his eye, fortunately didn't break his skull.

The collision occurred in February of 1949, on a foggy morning in the Chihuahuan Desert on two-lane Highway 80 in west Texas. L.H. Hogan, the driver of a westbound Greyhound bus, had unwisely passed the slow car in front of him. The bus weighed 20,000 pounds plus the weight of the passengers and their luggage and was doing about thirty-five mph. Hogan's eastbound '48 Caddy had no chance.

The key detail—both for Hogan's survival and in the tsunami of love and approval that was about to wash over him—was what he did a split second before impact. When the high headlights of the bus abruptly filled the interior of the car like a flash of lightning, Hogan shouted, "Look out!" and threw himself sideways, in front of his wife, Valerie. Valor or instinct? Both, probably. Diving hard to his right saved his spouse from harm and saved Ben from violent contact with the steering column, which rocketed into the car alongside the engine. As you could tell by looking at the wreck after they'd pulled him out of it, the steering apparatus would have impaled him.

"He saved my life," pale-faced Valerie said in the aftermath, and she kept saying it. The quote made the second or third paragraphs of hundreds of newspaper reports on the crash the next day and was repeated ad infinitum.

And in that moment, Hogan's image was transformed. But *just* his image. Circumstances change, sometimes very quickly, but it's debatable if people do.

Who was this brave man? Although he'd won thirteen tournaments in '46, seven in '47, and ten in '48, including the PGA Championship and the US Open, "Bantam Ben"—a nickname he hated—was a symbol of excellence and a respected sports figure but not an extremely popular one, nothing like Arnie and Tiger would become. He was also tough as a two-dollar steak, this one-hundred and-forty-five-pound battler with a thirty-seven-inch sleeve, the balance of a tightrope walker, a careful center part, and the fast-twitch muscle fibers of a gunslinger.

All his contemporaries agreed that the wins didn't make him happy, however. Something was eating at him.

Aided by his startling light blue eyes, Hogan owned and operated an intimidating, keep-away stare that made clear how he got one of his other nicknames—The Hawk. He scared people, which was a useful skill for someone who preferred to be left alone. He was an old man the few times we spoke in person, but I could agree with what 1964 PGA champion Bobby Nichols said: "He could look you in the eye and almost hypnotize you."

But at the same time, Hogan took pains to always be correct in word and deed. He sweated mightily over his correspondence, producing letters that could have been written by the most expensive and erudite attorney. Ditto the fit, finish, and muted colors of his clothes of Pima cotton, cashmere, linen, and good wool. Once a desperately poor boy, the wealthy man wore custom-made shoes both for the street and the golf course, size seven. He was fastidious regarding food. His manners were impeccable.

I suppose I was the first or at least the most obvious un-degreed psychologist to trace everything back to Ben's father, Chester. On the night of February 14, 1922, Chester pulled a .38 revolver out of his bag, turned it around, and shot himself in the chest, with nine-year-old Ben probably watching. A lot in Hogan's life from that point on—his distrust, the simmering anger, the stoicism, his burning desire to achieve—can be referred back to the grievous wound he was protecting. Maybe.

Author and suicide survivor Richard Rhodes wrote of his "empty, aching, longing expressed in little drips," in his book *A Hole in the World*. "I could be my own father, but I'd have to find my way across childhood first." Quoted here because Hogan never talked about it. Ben's father's self-murder was his closely held secret. Even Byron Nelson didn't know, and he both grew up and traveled the tour with Hogan for a while.

The loss of a parent is hard enough when the child has time to prepare for it and to say goodbye, but sudden death can cause permanent damage. According to the experts, boys are slower to move on than girls, who grieve more intensely. The physical fallout can be easily measured, writes Joshua A. Kirsch in a story for Fatherly.com, but "the psychological impacts are all but unpredictable."

Whether from his father's death or not, the burden of celebrity did not rest easy on Hogan's shoulders. The fish bowl did not suit the introvert. "What are you looking at?" he said to a father and son who were watching him hit bunker shots. Autograph hounds got the coldest of cold shoulders.

"I was riding in an elevator in a hotel, I think it was during a US Open," a man named Ed Preisler told me years ago. Preisler was a top amateur golfer from Cleveland. "My son, who was about ten, was with me. Hogan and [Jimmy] Demaret get on the elevator. I told my son that these were very famous golfers, that he should ask for their autographs. Hogan says, 'I don't give autographs.' Demaret played it perfectly. 'Come on, son, I can still write,' he says. I have no regard for Hogan as a person."

And Hogan had no regard for photographers. His one-hundred-watt smile and big gorgeous teeth lit up the day at the trophy presentation but shooters trying to get candids got The Look instead. Good thing the golf beat writer for the local paper—Dan Jenkins of the *Fort Worth Press*—got him, because Hogan's relationship with the notebooks had its ups and downs.

One of the downs occurred six months before the crash. While winning the Denver Open, Hogan gave great offense by running off to catch a train to the next tournament when he still had a chance to win this one. Sure enough, the leader, Fred Haas, Jr., stumbled to the finish and the absent Hawk had won. Dudgeon in Denver soared a mile high.

Hogan's walkout climaxed a long series of unpleasant incidents in which the Hershey prima donna let one and all know that he is good—and he knows it. He refused flatly to appear in Wednesday's clinic. Asked by a respectful radio reporter to say a few words, he refused flatly. With oaths, he refused a most reasonable request of photographers who sought

to snap him along with the obliging Haas and co-operative Cary Middlecoff . . . He refused a seven-year-old an autograph, saying, "Go away."
  —Rocky Mountain News, **August 23, 1948**

But that was then, before he saved his wife's life, nearly losing his own.

Letters to America's new hero arrived by the hundreds at the Hotel Dieu hospital, a hulking redbrick edifice in downtown El Paso. There were usually reporters around, covering the twists and turns in his slow recovery, especially his emergency surgery for blood clots. He lay there for fifty-nine days. From his window he could see the winter sun set on the mountains in Mexico and hear the bells from St. Patrick Cathedral. At the train station on the day Mr. and Mrs. Hogan went home, photographers snapped a shockingly emaciated patient strapped to a gurney. The man wore a brave smile; his wife a weary, worried look.

He rehabbed like mad.

His comeback tournament, the one that cemented his legend and that recalls Tiger at Augusta in 2019, occurred a year and a half after the crash. With a sweet one-iron on the seventy-second hole and despite cramping legs, Hogan won the 1950 US Open in a thirty-six hole, three-way playoff. Very dramatic stuff. You can read about it in *Hogan,* David Barrett's *Miracle at Merion,* or James Dodson's *Ben Hogan: An American Life.*

Woods endorsed Rolex; Hogan, Timex. Tiger had two years at Stanford; Ben dropped out of R. L. Paschal High after the ninth grade and he hadn't been going much before that. Woods had an involved father, to put it mildly, but Hogan . . . Tiger was a prodigy who won six times in his first fifteen months as a pro, including the '97 Masters. Ben didn't win enough money to mark his ball in four failed attempts to make the tour and he didn't win his first tournament until 1940, when he was twenty-eight (he won a team event in '38). He took the '46 PGA Championship for his first major.

But William Ben and Eldrick Tont had this in common: both men, while in the midst of almost unprecedented success, scrapped their carefully built golf swings. It was a necessity in Hogan's case, given the injuries he sustained in the car accident. But Tiger . . . after he won the '97 Masters so convincingly, and won again in his next event, the GTE Byron Nelson Golf Classic, and again a few weeks later in the Western Open, he decided he hated his swing. Hated it. Videotape told him he was not achieving the aesthetic beauty he sought, and that he was a little wild off the tee.

No, he told Butch, he didn't want incremental change, he wanted a total re-model. He'd be setting old adages on their ears: for Tiger, it wasn't how many, it was how. It wasn't broke, but he fixed it anyway.

Authors Benedict and Keteyian find compulsion and compulsion's cousin, anxiety, in this. Tiger's "quest for total control," they say, also helps explain his slavish devotion to the gym and to the practice tee. Or maybe that's just genius for you; it's "the infinite capacity for taking pains," as the old expression goes, like Edison finally inventing the light bulb after one thousand failed attempts. Said another way, Tiger had an infinite capacity for working his ass off.

Changing golf's most successful swing seemed strange but there were a lot of other things about the new sheriff a lot of us just didn't get.

Like: how could this most thrilling performer be *so boring* when his lips were moving?

It's difficult, I assume, for athletes to say anything interesting. In the over-heated moments after the game, the mental transition from competition to analysis must be arduous. We get that. No one is surprised when the comment offered is a repetition of what the coach said before tipoff or kickoff. "We knew we had to stay aggressive/win the fourth quarter/keep our poise/avoid big mistakes/not order the nachos"—whatever.

The other fallback, the one Tiger used, was the time-honored rhetorical device of humans who are forced to talk when they have nothing to say: the cliché. Before the tournament or after the round, Tiger could be relied on to communicate almost nothing at all, sometimes quite artfully. Someone—probably Earl, who considered himself a master media manipulator—had told him to treat the pens and microphones as the enemy and not as a means of credible free publicity. Hiding stuff from the press—hiding stuff from everybody—was part of his identity.

Here's an example of an unenlightening utterance from Tiger's Phoenix Open presser one year: "The field we have assembled here, obviously are some of the top players in the world, and with that in mind, obviously there's going to be some great play and hopefully I can be right up there."

Obviously. If he'd told us of his firm plan to continue putting his pants on one leg at a time, no one would have been surprised.

I became convinced that the fault was partly ours, his questioners. Better interrogatories would draw him out, I thought. Instead of "How happy were you with your game today?" I'd ask him about the interplay of Buddhism and Baptist-ism in his house when he was a kid. Did he and his mom care about or talk about the Thai royal family—King Rama IX and the others? (The diminutive Mrs. Woods, the former Kultida Punsawad, was from Kanchanaburi, Thailand, as you probably know.) I'd posit that caddie programs would get golf more new players than the First Tee ever would, and that no one should imitate Tiger's swing unless they were also going to work out like him—what's your take on that, Tiger? Ever had your aura analyzed? Your palm read? And so on.

In 2000, from out of nowhere—well, New York City—came a chance to test my theory on de-boring Tiger. There was a book in need of an author, the man on the phone said. It was all set up: the agent, the publisher, the title, the money.

There had been a writer for this project, but for reasons kept hidden from me, the other guy was out. Did I want to write a book entitled *Chasing Tiger*?

It was a crowded field; in his first three years as a pro, more than fifty Tiger-centric books had been published and the number appeared to be growing every hour. Earl added a couple: his sharp appetite for money and credit had compelled him to produce two volumes that he didn't actually write, *Training a Tiger* and *Playing Through*. On the other hand, the title and premise of the proposed book seemed spot-on: professional golf had become an exciting, discouraging pursuit of just one guy. Tiger was the mechanical rabbit at the dog track. But wait a minute: where was Tiger regarding *Chasing Tiger*? Did he know about it? Would he co-operate—would I get access? Yes and yes, the agent said, and the deal was done.

Thus, it was my fate to travel all over this great country for half of 2000 and half of 2001, in pursuit of the uncatchable. Forthwith, a few highlights:

1. Tiger winning the 2000 US Open at Pebble Beach by fifteen. Fifteen.
My most vivid memory of the week was watching sixty-year-old Jack Nicklaus walk past. Outlined against the infinite blue Pacific and under a clear blue sky, the sun caught the Bear's still-blondish hair. It was a poignant moment for me because my childhood hero was playing in his final US Open (he shot 73-82 and missed the cut), while Tiger was shooting 65-69 and

taking a six shot lead into the weekend. It wasn't a torch-passing, exactly, but a reminder that the torch had already been passed, and that this new guy might actually be as good as my childhood hero, if not better. This was a concept I struggled with.

Tiger didn't. As the other players were chasing Tiger, Tiger was chasing Jack. As everyone knew, Most Majors Won was Woods's white whale. On that Sunday night, as the new champ kissed the trophy, Jack led, eighteen to three.

2. A-Rod naked.

As months went by and my deadline clock ticked, Tiger's representatives seemed less and less interested in arranging a meeting. I kept reducing my ask from ten minutes to five to three, and the questions from "a few" to whatever. Got nada. Asking his friends for insight seemed a logical way to get around the roadblock; one such was the Texas Rangers' new shortstop, Alex Rodriguez, the fabulous A-Rod, who'd be getting over $2 million a month to toil for the local nine.

Nita Wiggins, a friend and sports reporter for the Fox TV affiliate in Dallas, set up a meeting. I'd never been in a major league locker room before and was not hip to the interesting and illegal things the players were doing to improve themselves at the time.

As Nita and I waited at A-Rod's locker, I observed the super hero torsos on his shirtless or t-shirted teammates. "These guys must spend all their time lifting!" I said. "They're bigger than a football team."

The interviewee arrived only a minute or two after the appointed time. He disrobed; my companion turned her back. She'd had to put up with this kind of thing before.

But then he didn't re-robe. Didn't put on anything but an unhappy face. For reasons I couldn't fathom then or now, A-Rod was going to do our interview in the all-together.

It didn't go well. After some preliminaries, I got out my pen and a notebook and kept my eyes upstairs.

Q. What brought you and Tiger together? What's your bond?
A. It's because we've both gone through . . .
because we're both minorities (Rodriguez's parents are from the Dominican Republic).
Q. What do you guys talk about? Your sport or his? The pressures in your lives?
A. I'm not going to talk about our private conversations!

That was about it. I tried one or two more salvos, but the naked shortstop was through with me. He looked good naked, by the way—godlike, in fact—but like others in that locker room, he might have had some help. A-Rod tested positive for steroids in 2003.

3. Green Magma.

A visit to the HQ of Tiger's agency, IMG in Cleveland, was

most enlightening, thanks to Alistair Johnston, a Glaswegian who was nominally in charge of the most powerful entity in sports, and, not coincidentally, also Arnold Palmer's personal agent. Tiger's guy, Mark Steinberg, sat in the office next door but was unavailable for comment, a disappointment but no surprise.

No matter: "Steinie," as Tiger calls him, had had little to do with the staggering $40 million deal with Nike or the other endorsements that made Woods a very wealthy man at age twenty-one. Besides, Arnie's journey as a celebrity pitchman connected directly to Tiger's—same sport, same agency, and some of the same people, including Johnston.

Since the earliest era in the funny game of endorsements, when Harry Vardon credited his great success to 3-in-One bicycle and gun oil, anyone might endorse anything. Sam Snead appeared in ads for Lucky Strikes, Viceroy, and Chesterfield cigarettes, for example—and he didn't smoke. Tiger endorsed Buick but did anyone think he took a Regal to the club? He drove a Porsche.

Arnie recommended we all try Green Magma, which sounds like a horror film starring Jeff Goldblum and Jennifer Lawrence but was actually concentrated barley juice powder "that meets your nutritional needs *naturally*." In a very long career of pitching things, Palmer pitched a lot of things, from Coca-Cola to coal.

To ketchup. In the quaint old days, someone asked Arnie to sit at a table and hold a knife and fork as if cutting into a steak and look pleasant and we'll pay you five hundred bucks. Sure, he said; a child of the Depression, Palmer found it hard to say no. In the resultant ad, next to "star golfer Arnold Palmer" stood a model portraying a waitress holding a bottle of "richer, thicker Heinz." But that sort of penny ante business stopped once Arnie got rolling with IMG.

Tiger's portfolio, by contrast, is far smaller but each company pays him far more. Any other comparisons, Mr. Johnston?

Palmer and Woods, he said, "are analogous in that both took golf to a new demographic. Arnold took it outside the country club and to Europe. Tiger's appeal is to an age group and an ethnic group. He's taken golf 'low,' that is, to ethnic minorities. He's made the game cooler to them."

Arnold's brand emerged over time. "Quintessential American hero," said Johnston. "Successful. But Tiger comes from a generation that does not expect to work for thirty years for recognition. A very impatient culture. They want accomplishment and riches now."

4. Walking along with Himself in 2000 at the Memorial—which he won—and the 2000 PGA Championship—which he won—and others I forget.
I didn't see much that you didn't see. Before he weight-lifted his torso into the shape of a martini glass, up-close Tiger looked like a track athlete or a wide receiver; muscles hung on a thin frame. When a shot went astray, he swore like the son of a Green Beret, as you know. Mostly he maintained an

eerie calm. I marveled at how non-reactive he was to pressure or to the hubbub around him. I envied the clarity of his vision of the perfect shot and then his ability to execute it.

Caddie Steve Williams—he'd replaced the much more benign Fluff Cowan—reminded me of a security guard at the mall. A couple of times the Kiwi cowboy glared at me as if I'd just shoplifted a pair of sunglasses.

"He's kind of majestic, an awesome presence," someone who was seeing Tiger for the first time whispered in the gallery in Houston. "He's like royalty."

5. Pixels.

Sometimes I hiked along from inside the ropes, which provided a clearer picture of his fans: compared to the other players, Tiger's gallery was the newest to the game and therefore the least knowledgeable, the loudest by far, the most tattooed and pierced, and the most likely to run to the next shot after Tiger hit this one and who gives a damn if it bothers the other players. Tiger endorsed Nike and they endorsed Tiger, by buying clothes and shoes with the swoosh. "I am Tiger Woods" may not have been literally true but it wasn't just a slogan, either.

"Hey, get out of the way!"

"That's bullshit. How come you get to walk in there?"

I heard those and similar comments more than once. Just doing my job, I told the enthusiastic patrons, and got down on one knee to keep from blocking anyone's view.

It didn't occur to me then how many gamers there must be in a Tiger gallery. The *Tiger Woods 99 PGA Tour Golf* computer game for PlayStation was a hit for its producer, Electronic Arts, and they put out another very successful Tiger Woods PGA Tour game annually until 2013, when Rory became the cover boy. One innovation—the three-click swing method—was part of its addictiveness, I'm told. One thing the game didn't have was a pain in the ass sportswriter blocking the view.

6. McVeigh executed.

The 2001 US Open at Southern Hills in Tulsa was my last stop on the Tiger train. If Woods would do the heretofore unthinkable and win his fifth major in a row, it'd be a hell of a final chapter for my book. But melancholy invaded my mood on Monday, June 11, the day they strapped the Oklahoma City bomber to a gurney in the federal prison in Terre Haute, put a tube in his right leg, pumped in pancuronium bromide, and everyone in Oklahoma said, good riddance.

But things picked up, and big fun was had. On the night before the first round, and for one or two nights thereafter, my friends Dan and Gaylen and I were invited for cocktails at a beautiful home in the hills above Tulsa. I remember the magnificent view, and a drinking game involving wine corks, and that Tiger was renting the house next door. Honest.

"What's he like?" asked Kim, our hostess, a massage therapist.

I looked to my right, where behind a hedge and some trees, Tiger was doing . . . something. "Beats the hell out of me," I replied.

"He won't talk with you?"

"Hey, Tiger! Come have a drink!" one of the comedians in our group yelled into the soft night air. "Hey Tiger, let's have a putting match! Hey, Tiger!"

Kim revealed that she'd seen her famous temporary neighbor in the Ten Items or Less line at the Albertsons down below. He'd bought bubble gum, then climbed into an SUV with darkened windows. I made a mental note.

It's come down to bubble gum, I thought glumly. The promised access had not materialized and the determined blandness of my subject's public pronouncements rarely moved my pen across my notebook. I'd chased Tiger and caught . . . what? My book was discursive. Even I didn't like it. The planes hit the towers while I was in the middle of writing it.

Someone wrote—probably John Garrity in *Sports Illustrated*—that with our collective lack of insight into the man of the hour, we'd entered "The Leaden Age of Sports Writing."

"In fifteen years on the Tiger beat for *S.I.* I got exactly ten minutes of his undivided attention," Garrity recalls. "Let's see . . . I met him for the first time after a practice round at the LA Open when he was sixteen. 1992. He was great. He and Earl were absolutely, perfectly normal. They were going out for pizza later and Tiger was excited about having a new puppy."

The world turned quite a few times before Garrity got his next and last shot in 2007, when he was one of a scant handful of journalists invited on board one of Nike's Gulfstreams for a publicity tour in honor of the golf division's new driver, the Sumo. You may remember it as the one with the bright yellow treatment on the sole and back. The Nike people asked the writers to please remember to mention the Sumo's MaxBack technology in their stories, which delivers a lower and deeper center of gravity, low spin, and high launch. It was a good club.

The journos, Team Nike, and Team Tiger boarded at a private airfield near Portland and landed in El Segundo on Santa Monica Bay in Los Angeles County.

"Tiger was waiting for us there," says Garrity. "The idea was that he'd hit a ball with a Sumo down the runway and set the world's long drive record but he missed the runway with his first two shots. 'I'd never use a driver like this,' he said" (meaning the club was not set to his specs).

After Tiger hit, they made the writers get back on the plane. One by one, each was led into a little conference room in the little airport office for an interview with Mr. Woods that would last ten minutes. Exactly ten minutes. Garrity decided to focus his questions on business.

"Tiger was at the end of the table. A representative of Nike's communications team sat in a chair by the door.

There was a wall clock above our heads, like in a school," says Garrity. "I wasted thirty seconds with pleasantries. I was in mid-question when the minder said 'time.' I wasn't surprised. It was a very controlled environment. There was no way to ask a personal question. He'd almost certainly end the interview if you did."

The writer asked the subject where he was getting his financial advice. Tiger mentioned this billionaire and that, and a sheikh. Not Palmer, Nicklaus, Player?

"No," said Tiger. "Look at the mistakes they made."

The recently retired Garrity, one of the best-ever writers on golf, had a great ability to put his subjects at ease. He teased out two very interesting statements from The Enigma:

Regarding his various new ventures—including a golf course design firm—Tiger said, "I need to do all this to make sure I can support my family and secure their future."

That seemed a little hard to believe. To Garrity "it sounded like a phrase from an insurance salesman." People were wondering back then if Tiger was a billionaire yet. He's worth about $800 million nowadays.

Near the end of their talk, Tiger volunteered a truer statement: "I am by nature a control freak."

As the interview itself had demonstrated.

Garrity said thanks to the control freak and walked back toward the plane, passing the next interviewer on the way. One of whom absolutely amazed him. "He's this California writer who did their website and who for years was our source when we really needed something from Tiger but couldn't get it. What was his name . . . Mark Soltau. He's Mr. Tiger—but even he takes the ten! It turns out he had no more relationship with him than we did."

The jet hopped around the country and all the writers had to stay on board, all the way to Teterboro, New Jersey. They'd had to travel the entire country to get their ten with Tiger.

Fifteen years walking the Tiger beat informed two books by Garrity. *Tiger Woods: The Making of a Champion* is OK, pretty good. But *Tiger 2.0*, a collection of some of Garrity's best stuff in *Sports Illustrated,* is highly recommended. There's just one Tiger story in it.

And fifteen years of experience with one subject yields an informed opinion. "A pathological narcissist," Garrity says. "All of his human relationships were transactional. If you couldn't help him achieve his goals, he had no use for you. He'd walk past and look right through you. Versus Phil, who'd stop and ask, 'How's the wife?'"

On the other hand—going back to my time in the barrel: 65-69-71-67, 67-66-67-69, 66-67-70-67, and 70-66-68-68. Those were Tiger's scores in winning the 2000 US Open at Pebble Beach, the 2000 Open Championship at the Old Course, the 2000 PGA Championship at Valhalla in Kentucky, and the 2001 Masters—the Tiger Slam. That was eloquent. That was electrifying. For the first time, someone held all four of golf's modern majors simultaneously. While in the midst of that supreme effort and accomplishment, Tiger didn't owe me or anyone else introspection. He wasn't wired that way.

How *was* he wired?

Although looking at Earl doesn't answer every question about turn-of-the-century Tiger, his influence seemed great indeed, and each said the other was his best friend. Yes, Arnold Palmer followed his father into professional golf—as did David Duval, Davis Love III, Curtis Strange, Bill Haas, and Young Tom Morris—but Earl did more than just provide an example of a career. He made Tiger his career.

In 1988, when he was fifty-six and his son was thirteen, Earl quit his job in the defense industry in order to go full-time as a helicopter parent. IMG enabled this with a $50,000 annual salary for Earl to be its "junior golf scout," with a wink-wink understanding that when the time came to pick an agency, the Woodses would look no further.

In the second full year of the deal, at the 1990 US Junior Amateur at Lake Merced Country Club in San Francisco, Earl demonstrated how he acted in this world and how he stretched his dollar.

"Tiger was pretty much the best player, although he was only fourteen," recalls Dr. Al Oppenheim, an Internal Medicine physician, scratch golfer, and member at the club. The kid from SoCal made the semi-finals but barely answered the call to the tee for his match, according to Oppenheim, so sick was he from nervousness that someone had to coax him out of the restroom. The other boy won on the sixteenth.

Earl and Tiger were back at Lake Merced two years later for Sectional Qualifying for the US Open. And as they'd done two years before, they stayed at a member's house. So, no hotel bill. No anything bill. No tips. And, unfortunately, no gratitude.

Tiger and Earl had a saying that illustrated their us-versus-them attitude, said when they'd put the trophy in the car: "We came, we saw, we won, we got the fuck out of town!"

"America's guests," Oppenheim says. "They assumed we'd buy them breakfast, lunch, dinner, and alcohol for Earl every day, for both tournaments. Which we did. But they were most unappreciative. They never *once* said thank-you.

"I was walking down seventeen with Earl and I said, 'You and Tiger make an awesome team. It's too bad you won't be around to see his ultimate success.' Because I'd seen him eat and drink like a pig and smoke like it was going out of style. I found out later that he was really pissed at me for bringing up his health.

"Earl was an asshole."

And so it went for Team Woods all through the amateur years and long after financial insecurity disappeared as an issue. Even while putting vast sums at risk at blackjack tables in Las Vegas, Tiger ducked the dinner check and tipped so poorly that he reached number one on an internet site's Ten

Worst Celebrity Tippers, an unreliable ranking to be sure, but still.

"He is cheap," said Charles Barkley, on an episode of *The Oprah Winfrey Show*, when the subject was his young friend the golfer. "What's the word white people use? Frugal. Tiger's very *frugal*."

The frugal superstar's lame excuse for his alligator arms—that were too short to reach his wallet—was that he never carried cash. The real reason had to be deeper than that.

Does Garrity's diagnosis hold water? Maybe. Narcissists don't mind spending other people's money because we're in their debt already, and they find it hard to say "thank you" for the same reason. Tiger checks the box on some of the other elements on the NPD (Narcissistic Personality Disorder) spectrum, including a strong need to exert control—over people, his press conference, his sand wedge. "Narcissists are control freaks" is a phrase you read over and over in the literature.

But if we think we've cracked the code by placing Tiger on a spectrum, we should think again. He's not that simple.

"A narcissist? No, I don't think so," says Jaime Diaz, who knows Tiger as well as—probably better than—any writer. "He's not like Trump, who needs constant affirmation. Tiger *never* brags. Never. Fame inhibited his maturation, so I'd cut him a lot of slack there. He was so scrutinized. I think when he was younger he put on a pose that was not his best self—cool, and older than his years. He wasn't. That explains his behavior with the *GQ* writer [who quoted the young man telling dirty jokes to young women].

"Among people he knows and trusts, he's good company. A good listener, and he's *so* knowledgeable about golf. But he'll always be an introvert. He prefers that the other guys tell the jokes.

"He'd had enough attention a long time ago. That's why he loved his two years at Stanford, because stardom there was based on academic achievement. Their hierarchy was 'who's the smartest kid?' not 'who's the best golfer?'"

What about Earl?

"I think his parents brought him up well, except for the 'genius' part," says Diaz, a Northern Californian whose lyrical pen made him a mainstay at *Golf Digest* for thirty years. He's a spoken word essayist now, on The Golf Channel. "Earl's pitch was always, 'Tiger is a once in a century talent, and we're giving you an opportunity to see him.'"

Another mitigator is that self-centeredness is baked into professional golf like flour in a cake. With no need to co-operate with a teammate or a coach, and with an agreeable valet and baggage handler (caddie) at his side in competition—who else is this game about but me, me, me?

Furthermore: extreme self-regard and lack of empathy seem to occur organically, like warts, in some people we could name. But Tiger had his attitude imposed on him by Earl and by the environment Earl helped create. The father was the grandiose one, not the son, who was simply grand.

Tiger's goal of supplanting Jack as the greatest major winner ever would seem to be over-the-top for anyone else but just look at what he's done! It's eighteen to tie and nineteen to win; he's at fifteen, and, possibly, counting.

As for his game face: Woods, Hogan, Gary Player, and others have gotten reverential commentary over the cocoon of concentration in which they played, but looking through people is not an unusual skill. Hundreds of thousands of urban commuters do it every day, as they go here and there on the subway and on the crowded streets, never making eye contact with anyone. Ditto the here-but-not-quite-here headphone wearers and cell-phone talkers on trains, planes, and at Starbucks.

Perhaps Tiger achieved such a deep dream state in competition that his trance persisted out in the real world. Or maybe he just didn't give a shit about people.

I ran this analysis past Peter Jacobsen. Like Diaz, he thinks it misses the mark. A U of Oregon diehard and a graceful and lucid TV golf announcer, Jacobsen won seven times on the PGA tour and twice more in the Senior division. He met the Woodses when Tiger was winning the Junior at Waverley, and they shared the dais at the dinner. They had first connected earlier in '93, when the sixteen-year-old played in his first tour event, the Nissan Los Angeles Open.

"It was Ernie Els, Tiger, and me," the Oregon Duck recalls. "I was immediately impressed by how well Tiger kept his eyes on the prize. He had the focus and the resolve to reach his goal, which was to be the best."

Three years later, when Peter was injured and Tiger needed a looper for his professional debut, Jacobsen loaned him his bearer, Michael T. "Fluff" Cowan. Through Fluff, Jacobsen and the Woods crew bonded. There were numerous dinners and phone calls amongst and between them all.

Cowan is a Mainer and sounds it, and a Deadhead, and looks it. "This kid hits shots unlike any I've evah seen," an amazed Fluff told Jake in a report from the front. Tiger called Uncle Peter that first week, too, to express his pleasure with two professional perks: the courtesy car and the no-charge buffet lunch in the locker room.

Woods and Cowan would win the '97 Masters together, but the professional relationship would last just two and a half years. "The money don't mean nothing to me," Fluff told a reporter before the '97 US Open. "I believe in the '60s. I don't believe in the '90s." But when he told another writer his financial arrangement with his new boss—a thousand a week and a ten percent commission on winnings—Tiger fired him. Fluff found his refuge looping for Jim Furyk and was on his bag when Furyk won the 2003 US Open at Olympia Fields Country Club outside of Chicago.

As for Earl, Jacobsen found him to be perfectly reasonable and not a hovering "tennis dad"—a fair point because Tiger moved out of hovering distance, to Florida, while Pops stayed put at the family home in California.

What about the way Tiger carried himself?

"Look, you don't have to pass a public relations test to

be a great golfer," Jacobsen says. "You just have to put twos, threes, and fours in the little boxes on the scorecard."

Tiger did exactly that and it was enough for a while. But one's wiring is important when dark forces gather and align to bring you down. Death, ego, and the fame machine knocked Tiger on his ass a decade or so ago, and a lot of the people who'd cheered for him now sneered at him. The indelicate phrase "shit storm" seemed invented for his new situation. Puritans and Calvinists came out of the woodwork and raised a din. Woods seemed suddenly to personify something or other, like pride goeth-ing before a fall, or Icarus, or King Lear. Media outlets specializing in the lurid enjoyed a series of feasts.

It wouldn't have been the same if he were, say, a hockey player. Golf holds itself out as the morally superior sport—and it may be—and it's committed to the idea that learning to play by its rules somehow nourishes "character" and that programs like First Tee create good citizens. Then the game's greatest player turns out to have a personal life based more on Hugh Hefner than Bobby Jones or Old Tom Morris. Along with other things and people, even Golf became furious with Tiger.

Name a celebrity in any field that ever had a more complete and humiliating disaster. And then a crippling injury.

Could the Comeback Kid come back from all this? How much could he take?

• • •

More than half a century ago, a couple of other champion golfers fought back from the edge of the abyss. Their stories and the people involved aren't similar to Tiger, except in their absolute refusal to give up.

One other thing characterizes all three: their—sorry, Lexus—relentless pursuit of perfection. If I may:

I am strongly opposed to both concepts. I am a huge fan of giving up—on a bad job, a bad marriage, the wrong goal, whatever. Quitting is so often the best option in life, much more often than sticking it out is. Recognizing a lost cause or a bad fit is in fact the soul of discernment and adaptability, a sign of nimbleness in one's life, and it employs a higher level of thought than "never give up."

And I despise the very idea of perfection, which is an anchor on human endeavor. Perfect is the enemy of done. Perfect is the disapproving voice telling you your physics grade could have been higher, your form on your *tour en l'air* in Act II could have shown more verve and balance, and you shot sixty-seven but you missed two putts under eight feet. Screw that, I say. Give it your best shot, get 'er done, and move on.

When a diesel truck repair school commencement speaker takes ill and they invite me to fill in, I plan to speak out forcefully against determination and perfection. Put that in your Juul and vape it, *grads*. I'll expect booing.

The point is, I simply can't comprehend the champions who keep practicing way past pretty damn good and who are never knocked off their path regardless of life's kicks to the groin. If there's a good bar in the next life, I would like to debate these issues with Tiger and a few others, like Skip Alexander.

Tall, affable Stewart Murray "Skip" Alexander could handle the academics at Duke University and he could also handle a golf club. A North Carolina boy from Durham, Skip was no blue-blood; he'd learned the game as a caddie at a little country course. Learned it so well that he won the North Carolina Amateur one year and the North and South Amateur at Pinehurst in 1941. The captain of the Blue Devils golf team graduated and then he just disappeared for the next four and half years, like so many others, and he didn't come home until the war was over.

He'd been in the Pacific, generally, and the Philippines, specifically. He didn't talk about it.

The mustered-out vet got an assistant's job at Lexington Golf Club, which is located about twenty miles south of Winston-Salem. There he learned the time-honored trick of the golf pro who can't remember a hundred new names but must act like he cares about each and every member: he just called everyone "Pard" or "Dude." "How'd you play today, Pard?' 'Dude, that sure was a good shot to eighteen."

In '47, his PGA apprenticeship complete, Skip arranged time off to play the tour. He virtually had to, because there was money laying out there on the ground, since whenever and wherever he played, his scores were so damn good. They stayed good; Alexander won the

National Capital and the Tucson Open in '48 and earned $2,000 for each; no fortune to be sure, but pretty good money when a new Buick Special cost $1,950 and the fuel to fill it was twenty-two cents a gallon.

The car-based post-World War II tour "was just a group of vagabonds," Skip would recall. "A close-knit group cuttin' up the same pie every week." You had to make the top ten every week to show a profit. Skip did.

Confirmation that Alexander had ascended to the top of American professional golf arrived when he made the Ryder Cup team in '49 and got to cross on the *Queen Elizabeth* and wear the same blazer and pants as Sam Snead, Jimmy Demaret, and Ben Hogan, the non-playing captain, who was still weak and shaky from his car accident. The Yanks won 7-5 at Ganton Golf Club in Yorkshire, England; Skip played in one match, the foursomes, and lost. But that didn't diminish the accomplishment of making the US golf All-Star team.

Things changed a bit for the next year's car/hotel/golf course marathon, because baby girl Bunkie—aka Carol Ann—had been born to Skip and Kitty, aka Kathleen. What the hell: they bought a suitcase that converted into a bed for the baby, and all three Alexanders hit the road. Despite the added stimulus, Skip killed 'em again. He won another tournament in '50 and a lot of cash and looked like a cinch to play in another Ryder Cup. That was going to be great, because the '51 Match was going to be held at Pinehurst #2, probably his favorite course. He'd won the North and South there, as we said.

In September of '50, after finishing sixth at the Kansas City Open, Alexander wanted desperately to get back to North Carolina for a quick visit before hitting the long road for an exhibition tour of South America. He couldn't find a flight, but an officer with the Civil Air Patrol offered to get him part of the way home; he had a small plane going to Louisville. As the tour's third leading money winner, Skip was a budding celebrity, and as a US Army Air Corps veteran—the CAP is the United States Air Force's civilian auxiliary—he had status. Sure, the big man said, I'd love a ride to Louisville. Thanks, Dude.

"Mayday, mayday." At about eight p.m., at six thousand feet, about 130 miles from Louisville, something went wrong with the gas tank on the Beechcraft T-7. The pilot switched to the auxiliary tank, but it wouldn't function, either. The four men aboard braced themselves; they'd try to make it the ten miles to the airfield in Evansville, in southern Indiana.

The silver-painted twin-engine prop plane flew low over the tents of striking International Harvester workers, then crashed tantalizingly close to the runway. Despite a crushed ankle and a broken leg, and the fact that he was on fire, Skip kicked a door open, got out of the plane, hopped a few agonizing paces, then collapsed. A savior named Ralph Reutter rolled him around to extinguish the flames and took off his still burning shoe and sock. Moments later, the back-up tank on the T-7 exploded, and the other three men were lost.

"He spent the next seven months in hospitals," says son Buddy Alexander, the 1986 US Amateur champ, and the coach of Florida Gators men's golf teams that won NCAA titles in 1993 and 2001. "They took so much skin from his rear end for grafts that his ass looked like a pair of madras pants."

Gasoline fire had incinerated half his ears. The visible areas of his patched and scarred skin had the rough look of spilled candle wax. But his hands . . . of the seventy percent of his body that had been burned, the man's poor hands looked the worst. As they'd burned, they'd blackened and curled almost into fists. The docs considered amputation early on, at least of the pinky fingers. As Skip would recall it, "My hands were all burned and now they're all skin-grafted. My fingers contracted so tightly that I didn't have any openings."

That the patient wanted to play golf again seemed like folly, but he had an idea. By cutting some tendons and removing some knuckles, perhaps the surgeons could open his hands into a semblance of a golf grip. It was worth a try. Alexander's friends at Wilson, his equipment company, made a miniature five iron with a regular grip for the surgeons to use as a template in the OR. On the head of the club they'd stamped "Little Dude."

One example of how much people liked and respected Skip: at the next Masters, the scarred man was escorted to a spot of honor: a chair in the shade of the long-leaf pines on the green, green grass between the twelfth green and the thirteenth tee, where no one is ever allowed but players and caddies. Old friends greeted him warmly, and some, at least, must have found a tear in his eye.

Based entirely or almost entirely on points he'd earned before the plane crash, Alexander squeaked in as the last qualifier for the '51 Ryder Cup team. It seems odd to us now, but back then—it didn't change until 1963—the format called for thirty-six hole foursomes matches on day one, and thirty-six-hole singles matches on day two, and let's have a drink. The '51 event had another wrinkle: an off day in the middle. The North Carolina Tar Heels football team had a home game against number-one ranked Tennessee. No one was going to watch golf that day. Heels fans didn't see that much football, either, as they fell 27-0 to the Vols.

Captain Sam Snead convened a meeting that night. Team USA led three points to one, so the outcome was still very much in doubt. It was time to talk strategy.

"Skip was disappointed that he didn't get to play the first day," Buddy says. "He thought if he played at all it would be in alternate shot." It was just as well. His hands probably couldn't take the beating, even if he only had to hit every other shot.

Captain Snead had a problem, though: one of his stalwarts, Dutch Harrison, had called in sick. How about you, Skip? Sam said. Wanna play? No way, objected Hogan, a man who knew from injury. He can't go thirty-six. Snead's strategy was plain enough: Alexander wouldn't have to play well, or even finish. He'd be the sacrificial lamb, because he'd have to go against the other side's best player, John "Gentleman John" Panton, a popular Scot who won almost everything Over There except the Open. Like Arnold Palmer, he'd have a drink named for him. A John Panton consists of ginger beer, bitters, and lime syrup.

The crazy-determined competitor gave it a go, but the thin, fragile skin on his hands didn't hold, and he bled badly—through bandages and then through two pairs of gloves and onto his grips. He even ran out of towels to bleed into near the end, and his legs ached. "Every time I played a hole I wondered if I could play the next," he said later.

That Alexander had even made it to the tee was a minor miracle; that he won, eight and seven, was a major one. It was the largest singles margin in Cup history. USA 9 ½ GB 2 ½.

That early November day was his final bit of glory. Alexander played in more tournaments in ensuing years but his career as a touring pro was over. He spent the rest of his working life as the golf pro at Lakewood Country Club, later re-named St. Petersburg Country Club, in Florida.

"It's a pretty similar story to Hogan, I guess, except that Skip was hurt a little worse," says his son. "But Dad didn't dwell on the career he lost. He always considered himself the luckiest man alive. Because he was alive."

That was Skip. Everybody loved Skip.

As perilous as his journey had been, Tiger's trip back to the top may have been just as tough. Let's see what we think after we look at it again.

PART TWO

Goodbye World

—

"It is every golfer's personal problem to master his judgements, yet I fancy none of us poor mortals will ever be more than mere toys for the devils inside us. Some days our judgements are uncannily correct and we may well-up with pride that at last, at long, long last, we are in command. But the next day we are back where we started."
—Five-time Open champion Peter Thomson in
The Secrets to Australia's Golfing Success, 1961

With everyone looking, and after some white lies and misdirection, Tiger went public with his new relationship. It wasn't the same as a movie star's ex bumping into the new girlfriend on a red carpet—but with the height of the profiles of the people involved, and the money and the egos, it was similar.

"Hank, good luck," said Claude "Butch" Harmon to Henry "Hank" Haney. "It's a tough team to be on. And it's harder than it looks."

The momentous meeting on the green carpet—the practice tee—at the 2004 Masters symbolized a profound change in the life of the new instructor of record. First of all, Haney could say ta to home and hearth in suburban Dallas. For the next six years, he would average 110 days per year of actual, physical, contact with Woods, at the boss's place in Florida, or on the road at a tournament—never, as far as I know, at one of Hank's practice facilities in north Texas. Another one hundred or so nights there'd be a text exchange or a chat on the phone. After the merest preamble, about the NBA or whatever—the talk would be of Tiger's grip, Tiger's right elbow at impact, Tiger's toes at the top of the buffet line. When it was over, Haney calculated they had about 1,200 conversations on the one subject. Tiger was an astonishingly dependent student.

The pay for the new guy would be $50,000 a year. Peanuts. Less than peanuts, really, when you consider the cost of almost four months a year of air fares, rental cars, Egg McMuffins, and hotel rooms, and the human cost of being away from home all that time. Yes, Haney would get a $25,000 kicker when Tiger won a major—he'd win six of them on Hank's watch—but just being associated with the best player in the world was what made the deal worth it. Haney's fame, credibility, and hourly rate would skyrocket. He didn't feel underpaid.

But all was not one-putts and sand saves behind the scenes, far from it. From the start, the relationship between the choreographer and the prima ballerina was incredibly intense and complicated. Haney ultimately felt so demeaned that he quit.

"It's a tough team to be on," Butch had said.

Rule one for this crew: be humble. In his 2010 book, *His Father's Son*, author Tom Callahan revealed the proximate cause of Butch's dismissal: seems Earl and Tiger were watching golf on TV, when instructor Harmon came on, and used a plural pronoun to describe various dramatic golf moments. As in "we hit a cut six iron in there pin high" and "we really needed to get off to a good start today."

And Tiger turned to Earl and said, "*We?*"

The new team consisted of Steinie, Stevie, Keith, Hank, and Tiger. Steinie—Mark Steinberg, the IMG agent and BFF—fielded the offers and protected his man like a hen with one chick. His nickname among media types was Dr. No—as in no, we will not comment on the rumors, and no, you cannot have two minutes with Tiger, and no and no and no. Stevie—Steve Williams—had reportedly not seen eye to eye with Butch. The gung-ho Kiwi guarded the boss's body with great vigor in the golf course milieu and performed the caddie function confidently and competently. Keith Kleven, the owner and director of the D. Keith Kleven Institute of Orthopaedic (his spelling, the British one) Sports and Dance Rehabilitation in Las Vegas, was an expert in building strong bodies twelve ways, at least.

Two others you might have thought were primary players in 2004 but weren't were Earl and Elin, Tiger's fiancée. Earl had hung on as long as he could in his son's business life but now Tiger had the awesome power of IMG behind him and the tip of the spear in Steinberg. So Pops, with his generally iffy health, stayed home and lived a sybarite's life, paying the masseuse's bills with the money from his job as the head of the Tiger Woods Foundation. Ms. Nordegren was, and would remain, in a lead-lined, walled-off segment of her future husband's compartmentalized life.

"The toughest guy on the team was Tiger," Hank would write much later. "One misconception was that he knew more about the golf swing than any modern player. Though Tiger definitely possessed a great deal of knowledge, he'd proved that he didn't have enough to fix himself."

Hank would *write:* thank goodness that inquiring minds like ours compelled Haney to pen a memoir of his six years on the team. That his tenure began in high renown but ended in very dark days gives his narrative both structure and momentum, but *The Big Miss* wouldn't be the entertaining book it is without Haney's ghost, *Golf Digest* Senior Writer Jaime Diaz.

Diaz was in a tight spot when he was offered the job and he didn't accept it right away. Despite good money up-front and the potential for more based on sales—the publisher's dreams of a flowing stream of cash were realized when the book reached number one on the *New York Times* bestseller list—there were other considerations. One hit Diaz in the face the moment he took the deal: "It ended my relationship with Tiger. Permanently."

Even the tiniest bit of rapport with the biggest man in golf—maybe in all of sports—was gold to writers and broadcasters. This often resulted in a kid glove, let's-not-offend-Tiger, sweetheart press that was an insult to the First Amendment. Most reporters dared not ask real questions. Notable exceptions were Jimmy Roberts and John Feinstein.

And Diaz. His substantial interpersonal skills kept the often bored and over-cautious interviewee from clamming up or reciting another cliché. Diaz knew his stuff, he'd known the Woods family since forever, and Tiger's mom liked him. That helped.

"When Tiger's fame caused him to limit his time with writers, I took no offense," Diaz says. "[But] for nine years, I had a once a year interview with him for what we [at *Golf Digest*] called 'The State of Tiger.' It was demeaned as a 'house job' but I thought it was pretty good."

It was. The fifth annual installment, in 2005, for example, which coincided with the stock-taking of Tiger's thirtieth birthday, revealed at least one "I didn't know that" facet of the planet's greatest golfer's worldview. "It's hard to make the ball move," Woods said, meaning that it had become increasingly difficult to purposely curve the orb in a useful way. He missed the old days, before equipment "innovations" dumbed down the game. "You look at the old guys who were or are true shot-makers, like when I played with Lee Trevino at Bighorn and he blew my mind with some of the shots he hit. Then you look on tour and you ask, 'who are the true shot-makers? Who actually maneuvers the ball or does something different with it?' And there really aren't that many, if any, out here anymore."

If he ruled the golf world, Tiger said, he'd return spin to the ball, "so misses would be more pronounced and good shots more rewarded." He'd also disallow wedges with more than fifty-six degrees of loft, to restore variety to the short game. "Nobody hits half shots anymore," he said.

It was a "house job," Diaz said, because *Golf Digest* and Tiger had been affiliated since he'd turned pro. The genesis of their long, mostly good relationship went back to 1990. In an interview with the *Birmingham Post-Herald* before the '90 PGA Championship, the founder of the host club addressed a ticklish question about its membership. "I think we've said that we don't discriminate in every area except the blacks," said Hall Thompson, and thus was born the Shoal Creek Controversy. Virtually from that moment on, host courses for tour events and majors had to come clean about their membership policies.

"After Shoal Creek, we published a two-part series on discrimination at private clubs," recalls *Golf Digest* Editor-in-Chief Jerry Tarde. "We tried to get involved in a positive way in welcoming minorities into golf. We partnered with John Merchant [a black USGA official] and held a number of symposia with black golf leaders. One of them was named Earl Woods.

"Earl and I played golf, got to know each other. Fast forward through his son's six national championships, and there's this mad dash to sign him when he turns pro. Well, that's what we do. The best—Jack Nicklaus, and Seve [Ballesteros], for example—write for us. But George Peper [then the editor of *Golf Magazine, Digest's* rival] saw a chance to grab the best guy. Not only the best guy, but the new face of golf. There was a heated recruitment.

"I had lots of conversations with Earl during the '96 Masters. One night we went to a jazz club in downtown Augusta. 'I really need your help,' I said. 'Don't worry, I'll take care of it,' he said."

And he did. Tarde was pleased to observe that Tiger's face on the cover spurred newsstand sales like no one else ever had or ever would, but as time went on, Woods would find less and less time to be photographed hitting shots for the instructional pieces written by *GD* staffers Pete McDaniel, Guy Yocom, and Mark Soltau. This was a problem, because "how I hit the 'stinger'"—or the flop shot, or left-handed, or whatever—were the magazine's backbone.

The thirteen-year relationship ended in 2010—a mutual decision, and without rancor, says Tarde.

But Team Tiger's association with *Golf Digest* Senior Writer Diaz wasn't necessarily over. There was an informal understanding between the parties that Jaime would be ghosting Tiger's autobiography (which Tiger wanted to write as much as he wanted to eat sand, which is to say, not at all) and another instructional book. If Diaz wrote a memoir for Hank the Disgruntled Instructor, or if he allowed it to be too honest, would those opportunities disappear? Did IMG hold that possibility over Jaime's head before he took the

Haney book, or during the writing of it? Diaz won't say, but the other books didn't happen. For Diaz had helped Hank breach instructor/student privilege—which hadn't been a thing until this very moment, because who ever even gave a damn about the back-and-forth between any other pair?

The Big Miss—published in 2012, two-plus years after the Revelations—fascinated me, and I recommend it, but if I hear another reference to "swing plane," I'm gonna hit somebody. "Swing plane" was in all likelihood a contrivance of Anthony Ravielli, the portrait painter turned illustrator who created the images for the golf instructor's Bible, Hogan's *Five Lessons*. According to a chat I had with the writer, the late Herbert Warren Wind, a lot of times it was image first, then concept. Ravielli sketched a pane of glass with Hogan in the middle of it and teachers have been fussing over "swing plane" ever since. Hank and Tiger found value in the conceit that a pleasing geometry was the key to the golf swing, while most of us, *Hank*, could use instructional articles entitled "How to Win With Your Crappy Swing" and "Effective Choking." The perfection he and Tiger sought isn't germane to most of the rest of us, an under-examined concept in the world of golf instruction.

Haney, says Diaz, was a great collaborator. When the putative author is uncommitted, inarticulate, or lazy, the job of the ghost is monumental, but Hank came to the writing table with a detailed plan and a sense of mission. His motivation came from the feeling that he had been scapegoated in the down times and given scant credit for his role in the team's success.

The Big Miss would be sold as a "tell-all" book but was it really just a "tell-some?" What, Mr. Diaz, did you leave out?

"The publisher was always pushing for more personal stuff, such as anything about Elin," Diaz said. "And some people were disappointed that the book wasn't more salacious. [On the other hand] the criticism we got from golf pros was that it was too personal. We decided that anything affecting Tiger's golf was fair game. And I think we showed that his peace of mind and his self-esteem were really ruined because of what he did."

Reviewers invariably focused on the "popsicle incident," finding that it showed in frozen form Tiger's startling lack of interest in other people, or, perhaps, that it illustrated the tunnel vision of this particular elite athlete. You may remember: after long days on the practice tee at Isleworth—which was in easy golf cart distance from Tiger's front door in his fortified community in suburban Orlando—teacher and pupil often repaired to Casa de Tiger. After dinner, with the game on the big screen, Tiger would walk to his Sub Zero and withdraw a single sugar-free popsicle; I've always pictured an orange one. And that's it, that's all Tiger did. He'd suck and lick his 'sicle while Hank just watched. The oblivious host never offered a frozen treat to his guest—who wanted one but felt funny about asking.

Per *The Big Miss*, when Steinie told Hank that Tiger

considered him to be one of his best friends, the instructor was baffled. He thought but didn't say: I am?

The popsicle and other examples of Tiger's arrested development revealed in *The Big Miss*—such as his learned inability to pick up a dinner tab or to simply say thank you, and silences as sullen as a teenager's gloom—should be held up to some of the champion's very positive traits. He was a humble man, and a fair competitor and sportsman. He took his philanthropy very seriously (and endowed his causes generously). Only a few of his fellow tour players could claim to know him—Tiger didn't blend—but they liked him and respected the gutsy way he reacted to pressure. And they really liked the popularity he'd brought to the sport, which made them all a shit ton of money. Purses when he joined the tour totaled about $101 million; twelve years later, in 2008, the number was $292 million.

But first in Tiger's plus column must be his willingness to put in the reps. He earned every bit of his success. He worked his ass off.

What Hank mentally referred to as Tiger Days at Isleworth went like this:

> He would begin a typical [day] by waking up at six and working out until eight. After he showered and ate breakfast, we would meet on the practice tee at nine for ninety minutes of hitting balls. From 10:30 to eleven he would practice putt, then play as

many as nine holes on the course until noon. After a one-hour lunch break, we'd meet at one p.m. for an hour of short game work, followed by another ninety minutes of hitting balls. From 3:30 to 4:45 he'd play nine holes, and then return to the putting green until six. This would be followed by an hour of shoulder exercises before retiring for dinner at seven.

Tiger respected practice. It was sort of his church . . .

Those of us who have written prose poems about Hogan's work ethic—or the epic practice tee endurance of Vijay Singh, Trevino, Player, Tom Kite, and a few others—have given short shrift to Tiger, who didn't practice so much as he trained. As if he were in the military. As if winning the next tournament was a mission.

• • •

Not to go all Gary Smith on you, but let's imagine for a moment what it was like to be in Tiger's skin. Let's say it's mid-April, 2005.

Writer Smith's psychiatrist's couch style had a pure expression in his long, melodramatic profile for *Sports Illustrated* of heavyweight champ and heavyweight sociopath Mike Tyson—*in the second person.* "You take your pigeons out of their cages one at a time and let them fly away. You wish that you could fly, too"—like that. I can't do that.

The Sports Whisperer applied his affecting but kind of creepy style to the magazine's 1996 Sportsman of the Year essay, when Tiger was the honoree (he'd be named SI's S.O.Y. again in 2000). But back then Earl approached the microphone or the shade of a writer's attention like a drunkard reaching for a drink, and he was flying over the moon with predictions that his son—no mere golfer, that boy—would unite the nations. Really, Earl—nations? Yes, he said a second time, *the nations*. Tiger had relatively little to add; he was a fraction of the man he'd be a decade later.

Tiger is on his couch in this imaginary moment. He pauses, pensive, between watching a DVD of a documentary he's seen so often he has it memorized, and a shooting game he's played hundreds of times. He looks back a few days to the previous Sunday afternoon, when he was leading the Masters by one shot with three to play but was leaking so much 10W-30 that his engine almost seized. He'd hit a horrid pull hook on sixteen, the snow globe short hole with a reflecting pond between the tee and the green. He'd looked at Stevie.

"Where's that?"

"It's long left."

"What's over there?"

"I don't know. I've never been there. I've never looked there."

Tiger's ball has come to rest in an untenable spot. Lush rough behind his Nike TW One Platinum complicated the shot—a lot—except they won't let you call it rough at the

Masters: it's the "first cut." Also: people aren't people, they're patrons.

In the hush, while announcers Verne Lundquist and Lanny Wadkins murmur their analyses, Tiger immerses himself mentally into the challenge of the moment. He harnesses self-belief and discipline. He removes the inhibition of fear. He lofts his ball with flawless trajectory and perfect spin to a precise square inch of hard ground, and the ball rolls very slowly sideways down the hill toward the hole through the sun-dappled shade or the shade-dappled sun, the patrons' sound mounting with every inch. The ball pauses as if exhausted by its crawl down the slope before slipping over the lip and into the hole. The patronage roars and Verne Lundquist loses it ("Oh, wow!" Verne says, not exactly a call for the ages) as Tiger and Stevie hop around and punch the air. They attempt a high five but whiff.

But even right thoughts and controlled breathing don't help that much when your swing feels like it belongs to someone else's body, like hand-me-down clothes.

After his transcendent chip, Tiger hit his drive so far right on seventeen that his ball almost reached the fairway on fifteen. Bogey. On eighteen, he pulled his three-wood tee shot into the left *rough*—there, I said it—a miss of the fairway for the fourth time in the final five holes. Then he went way right with his iron shot, the Nike TW One Platinum splashing into bright white bunker sand, a pretty bad shot. "God. Dammit!" the competitor exclaimed, and the CBS-TV audio was clear as crystal. Another bogey, and a tie with the dogged, unlucky (he lipped out his chip on eighteen) Chris DiMarco.

But then Tiger executed three flawless shots for birdie on the first playoff hole—eighteen again—to beat DiMarco. Now he'd won the Masters four times.

The aftermath had not been the usual thing. He had a wife to hug, for one thing—he and the gorgeous former nanny had jumped the broom six months earlier, in a quiet, private ceremony in Barbados that had cost in the millions. Don't know what helicopter rental prices were but the Woods Forward Nuptials Team leased every known Barbadian chopper to frustrate the paparazzi air force. The Team also rented the entire resort where the nuptialization took place; that set them back one and a half million. Now here was the beautiful blonde Elin in hugging position, wearing designer shades and a red top to match his own customary Sunday battle dress.

Earl was not there for his traditional, lingering embrace. *That* was different. Instead he watched the TV in his hotel room, too weak to come to the course.

The aftermath of the aftermath *was* the usual thing. Steinie did his best but he couldn't keep out all the noise, all the grasping hands and expectant faces. And the media was *such* a pain. Celebrity is corrosive, Tiger finds, like a steady drip of acid onto his life. His privacy has vanished like fog in sunshine. Wherever he goes, all eyes are on him, which results in a feeling of being trivialized, as if he is a roadside attraction. *Hey look, there's Tiger! Stop the car, Kathy!* Arnold Palmer is the only other golfer in history who made people swoon when he entered a room, but Arnie always liked it. He'd shake the hand of the man interrupting his dinner, sign the autograph, smile, and mean it. But Tiger's personality and circumstance are far different from Arnie's. He has to invent his own path.

But while his life has changed, he hasn't. What makes him tick—which he has said over and over, and people still don't quite understand—is his desire to know what's possible. Is it *possible* to be the best ever? It was possible for Bobby Jones and Hogan and Nicklaus. Therefore, it is possible to exceed them.

And now Tiger mulls the *rewards* of being a global icon. Let's see: there's the jet, the yacht, this house, this couch, the dive boat. The V-VIP treatment in Vegas is very sweet. Elin? Marriage is . . . OK. Hank thinks her smile gets smaller and smaller each time he sees her. Maybe. Maybe a lot of things.

There are other lives he could live. It's possible.

Tiger picks up the remote. Presses play.

"In war there are no timeouts, no contrived popularity contests to decide life and death," says a somber voice over images of beaches, explosions, and green-painted warriors in camo firing automatic weapons. "This program is about the eighty-three young men of Class 234 and their six months long struggle to become US Navy SEALS in a training course called Basic Underwater Demolition SEAL Training, or BUD/S."

Navy SEALs: BUD/S Class 234 is a six-part, four-hour and twenty-minute documentary from 2002 depicting a brutal weeding out process. On a beach, a shivering, exhausted sailor has to hold a downward-facing dog pose while an instructor piles sand on his ass. Teams of seven pilot rubber boats into fifty-four-degree ocean water and into waves a surfer would love. The maybe-SEALs wipe out time after time. Then they do it at night. They run four miles on the beach trying and mostly failing to make the required time of thirty-two minutes or less. They hold heavy poles overhead until their arms shake and then they do it again. Some inhale water and almost die in underwater swimming exercises.

In "motivational timeouts" the candidates do hundreds of pushups, while an instructor sprays them on the head with a hose and yells. "You don't give into the pain, you adjust to it!"

Another exchange is a staple:

Instructor: You know what second place is, right?

Potential SEAL: First loser!

"The main lesson of Phase One: individuals cannot survive in wartime," intones the somber voice-over. "Class 234 must develop a trust in teamwork no matter how high the surf and how wet and cold they become. Trust in one another is the essential SEAL trait for survival."

That would be cool, Tiger thinks, to be part of a stealthy, violent, and anonymous team and not a lonely solo performer, which is what he is, despite the in-air-quotes "team" of Steinie and Hank and the others. Could he deep-six fame and golf and a $60 million mortgage and a $50 million (on its way to $100 million) annual endorsement income and the strictures of golf and of matrimony? Is *that* possible?

Now Tiger imagines the covert life in another way. He puts down the remote, puts on the headphones, and picks up the PlayStation controller. *SOCOM: U.S. Navy SEALs* is ready to play. It's "a tactical shooter game emphasizing stealth and slow pacing to complete the objective and neutralize the enemy." Per Wikipedia, "it's meant to simulate realistic combat." An expert in this area—my son John—says that *SOCOM: U.S. Navy SEALs* is pretty good and a little bit harder than the average game.

Yes, the special ops thing is a possibility, Tiger thinks, but he's not thinking clearly. What I think he thinks is that the rewards for his sacrifice and accomplishment are not great enough. Perhaps extreme self-indulgence can tamp down the emptiness. He has the perfect cover to fool his wife, to fool everybody. He needs to be out of town on business a lot, and he has his own jet, a Plutonium credit card, fame, great teeth, and, as would become clear, a gaggle of gals who wanted to share the ride.

He picks up his phone. He's getting a text. Jaimee.

• • •

Grim reality intruded on Tiger's fantasy life when his father died on May 3, 2006. Earl Woods passed away at his home in Cypress, California, in suburban Los Angeles, at age 74. It was an old 74, what with his diabetes, poor circulation, and heart problems. His prostate cancer recurred in 2004.

Obituaries reminded us that Earl Dennison Woods was born March 5, 1932, in Manhattan, Kansas, the last child of six. His father was a stonemason. He was orphaned at age thirteen, and in addition to Tiger, he was survived by his wife Kultida; three children from a previous marriage, sons Earl, Jr. of Phoenix; Kevin, of Los Angeles; and a daughter, Royce Woods, of San Jose, California.

A lot of information about the father of the prodigy became available postmortem. Little of it is flattering, especially his philandering, which Tiger knew about and hated. Tarde of *Golf Digest* offers an informed and funny summing up:

"Regarding Earl: I am reminded of that wonderful exchange in *Casablanca* between Bogart and the young girl Annina. She says, 'Monsieur Rick, what kind of man is Captain Renault?' And Bogart replies, 'Oh he's just like any other man. Only more so.'

"We're all flawed, and maybe that's being too kind to Earl. I knew him as a friend—he was loyal, caring, funny, and pretty damn smart. We all have a special respect for people who served their country in the military. He did two tours of duty in Vietnam, the second with U.S. Army Special Forces. There's a part of Tiger that was always trying to measure up, I thought."

James Marcus, writing in the *New Yorker*, was eloquent

in describing the hole in his own life following the death of his father: "We were a religious sect consisting of two people. Now half the congregation was gone." To some degree that also applied to Tiger. At the bare minimum, he'd lost his best friend.

Haney was impressed by Tiger's composure when he eulogized his father at the Tiger Woods Learning Center, in Anaheim, which had been opened three months before.

Then what, now what? How would his father's death affect Tiger? Lives are blends of things, like melting Neapolitan ice cream, and events overlap and intersperse. We could organize a look at Tiger's journey in the years just before and right after Earl died by separating it into three sections: the golf, the SEALs, and that other thing. But these three activities did not happen sequentially; they swirled together to make his one life. That he kept all three of these heavy balls in the air seems incredible now.

Although he kept it hidden behind his poker face, surely Tiger grieved, and felt hurt and disrupted, but look at how he played! A couple of months after Earl passed, his son won the Open Championship at Royal Liverpool, and *then every tournament he played in for the rest of the year.* During this six-in-a-row win streak was another big one, the PGA Championship, at Medinah. It was his twelfth major win.

On the eighteenth green at Royal Liv, Tiger's emotions overflowed. "[He] fell into my arms and wouldn't let go," recalled Caddie Williams in his book, *Out of the Rough.* "I moved instinctively to separate from him—his victory hugs were traditionally short and sweet—but as I tried to break free his embrace tightened and I realized this wasn't the Tiger I knew. He was sobbing uncontrollably. I'd never seen him like this—ever."

In the hugging department, at least, Stevie would have to stand in for Earl.

Tiger won eight times in '06. Got seven more in '07 including the PGA Championship again, this time at Southern Hills. His adjusted (for golf course difficulty) stroke average in '07 was—more italics, please—*67.79*. That tied Tiger's 2000 for the lowest number ever (Nelson averaged 68-point-something in his big year, 1945; adjusted average is a new thing).

But stats blur the vision. The superlatives mount and lose their meaning. I enjoy thinking of Tiger in another way, as a young man in a Hootie and the Blowfish t-shirt and a backward-facing ballcap. He's showing his tombstone teeth and taunting his elders, who are in rocking chairs, and wearing lap blankets, flannel, dandruff, and thick glasses. And they don't hear well, so their voices are loud:

Tiger: Knock, knock, Sam Snead and Jack Nicklaus.
Sam Snead and Jack Nicklaus: (In unison) WHAT?
Who's there?
Tiger: Watcher.
Sam and Jack: WHAT? Watcher who?

Tiger: Watcher asses. Because I'll be taking Sam's record for most-ever wins eventually; it's your eighty-two to my sixty-five. Jack's major record, too. It's eighteen to thirteen now. By the way, I'm only thirty-two. Watch. Your. Asses!

It seems a shame to merely summarize Tiger's magnificent golf in these glory years, especially his unforgettable ninety-one-hole win in the 2008 US Open at Torrey Pines. You remember: the angels sang that week for Rocco Anthony Mediate, a sunny gent from wild Western Pennsylvania, who played the game with a bad back and an unlovely but functional golf swing that had won five times on the tour. In other words, Rocco Anthony Mediate could really play when he was on, and he was on. Tiger tying him after four rounds was remarkable, because he was getting by on only one anterior cruciate ligament, half the usual allotment, and he had a couple of hairline cracks in the tibia, too. A post-Masters surgery for "cleaning up" the troublesome left knee had revealed the serious structural problems. Woods walked as if he had spear grass in his socks that week and the mere act of following through delivered jolts of pain. This was Tiger's "Hogan at Merion" moment.

Midway through the second round, just before Destiny made Tiger its child and put the hole in the way of a chip or two and lots and lots of long, long putts, he swung at a ball and it hurt him so much he seemed near tears.

"Is it really worth it, Tiger?" Stevie asked.

"Fuck you, I'm winning this tournament," replied the one-legged golfer.

Rocco spoofed Tiger in the eighteen-hole playoff, by showing up in a red shirt and black trousers. "Nice fucking shirt," Tiger said during the warm-up, and he was miffed, not joking. "Last clean one I had," replied Rocco. Or was it?

In any case, neither Woods nor the moment could intimidate Mediate; they played eighteen more holes and tied again. Tiger won the sudden death hole with a par and then he was off to see his surgeon.

His knee and leg trouble had become chronic. While a freshman student-athlete for the Stanford Cardinal, Tiger had endured his first operation on the union of the thighbone and the shinbone, for removal of scar tissue and a benign (non-cancerous) cyst, the cyst being a little bag of joint fluid that formed on the back of his knee. It formed because of persistent leaking caused by chronic inflammation due to persistent hard swinging at golf balls. The damn thing returned, as they often do, and Tiger had to have another cystectomy in 2002. With that one big joint in mind, he decided he had to change his swing again. It had to be stressed less, somehow. That had been Hank Haney's original charge when they got together in '04: find Tiger a new, knee-friendly stroke.

Maybe his workout was partly to blame; perhaps it had acquired a new edge and intensity. In his admirable zeal to get stronger and win more golf tournaments—or from a preening self-regard and desire to look good for the other gender—Tiger had been exceeding by orders of magnitude the weight of the weights his trainer, Keith Kleven, preferred. Kleven advocated high reps. Tiger thought moving very heavy weights as quickly as possible was best for him.

Perhaps his swing—not just the frequency of use but the way he swung—led to injury. Tiger's technique, especially with the driver, included a move called "posting up," which is straightening the left leg at or just after impact. In the right hands, posting up increases the distance the ball will fly, but a straight leg doesn't absorb shock too well, according to my ski instructor, so the bump from a mogul or the stress of weight transfer in a golf swing radiates into the knee ligaments, the spine, and the neck.

Hence, Tiger became a (lowercase) wounded warrior. From 2007 up to and including 2019, except for one year, he had minor to crippling injuries *every year*, and seven surgeries.

SEAL training could also have played a part in his physical breakdown. Tiger trained on an honorary basis, but it was real training, and therefore dangerous. He got badly bruised on the thigh by a rubber bullet and once got kicked hard in his already sore knee. Along with real Sea, Air, Land virtuosos of the killing arts, he jumped from planes, practiced his hand-to-hand combat skills, simulated urban combat, and fired various weapons at various targets. Unsurprisingly, he proved to be a good shot. On his own, he ran and ran in combat boots, a weighted vest, and camo. He was already an expert diver; he was super-fit. His mental strength was through the roof. Tiger had all the attributes of a successful candidate, except one.

In 2007, when he was thirty-one, the erstwhile golfer trained on six occasions with the SEALs. Caddie Williams had known about his obsession for years; after a poor showing in the 2004 US Open, Tiger had pulled their car to the side of the road. "Stevie, I think I've had enough of golf," he said. "I'd really like to try to be a Navy SEAL."

A SEAL? Steinie was incredulous. Haney was dubious. "Aren't you too old?" the teacher asked Tiger one day. Good question, because according to navy.com, "Navy SEAL recruits must be between the ages of seventeen to twenty-eight. There are some waivers for men ages twenty-nine and thirty that are available for very qualified candidates. These applicants must prove to the Navy and Navy SEAL community that they are worth the investment."

"It's not a problem," Tiger replied. "They're making a special age exception for me."

We wondered what a guy who'd been there and done that thought. Would Tiger have been able to make it through the training? Would he have been someone you'd want to fight beside?

"Yes," says Aaron Silton, a former Marine Corps Raider. Raiders are the rough equivalent of SEALs, Rangers, and Green Berets; an elite and especially lethal military force. "Tiger can do whatever he wants to do. Being a special operator is no more than a mindset. In training or on a mission, it's not being able to quit. And Tiger has no quit in him."

Woods wanted to transition from golfer to warrior; Silton did the opposite. His unlikely path to the first tee started in a firefight in a dusty little village in southwest Afghanistan in September 2009.

He'd dispatched a dozen enemies, probably more, when a bullet fired by a Taliban sniper from a Dragunov rifle found Silton's head. The finger-sized shell tunneled through his cheek, teeth, tongue, and neck before lodging in the butt stock of his machine gun. Fellow Marines pulled Silton out of the hot orange sand and the bee-infested thorn bush he'd had fallen into, but too roughly—severely dislocating his shoulder. It got worse: on the operating table in Kandahar, Silton suffered a massive stroke. And a harried medic needlessly stuck surgical staples into his scrotum. *Damn.*

What was the worst part of his life after that? The surgeries, the months in bed with a jaw wired shut, the slurred speech, the anger, the obsession with returning to Afghanistan to blow away the motherfucker who'd shot him? Or was it the PTSD? After months in Walter Reed National Military Medical Center—where he became friends with comedian Jon Stewart, a good-hearted man for visiting wounded vets—Aaron was transferred to Camp Pendleton in San Diego for more months of rehab. He and his wife lived off base. It didn't go well. Silton wouldn't, couldn't leave home without his Remington Tango 1-MT knife on his hip.

"Dinners were OK," Silton says. "Parties, no. I had a short fuse. I could get to physical violence very quickly."

Recalls Tiffany, his wife: "We had to stop going anywhere."

Some version of that could have been Tiger's life if he'd cast aside wealth and celebrity in favor of serving his country by fighting its wars. There had been a recent example of a professional athlete doing exactly that. Pat Tillman, the hard-hitting strong safety for the Arizona Cardinals, had been so outraged by the attacks on 9/11 that he vowed to do something about it. He played well during 2001's sad football season, his fourth, so well that the team put a three-year deal on the table for a million point two annually, roughly doubling his pay. Instead Tillman kept his promise, enlisted in June 2002, and became another kind of bad-ass, an Army Ranger, and was subsequently deployed to Iraq and Afghanistan. He was killed by friendly fire in April 2004. Jon Krakauer's book on Tillman's journey—*Where Men Win Glory*—should not be missed.

The punchline to Silton's story: One day in rehab, someone handed him a set of golf clubs—he'd never hit a ball before, except for some home run swings with his high school buddies at a driving range back home in suburban Boston. "This game sucks," the Raider said. "Why would anyone play it?" But the thrill he felt with every solid strike during this second shot at golf fueled his epic return from the brink.

Today the guy with a bullet through his head is a golf

instructor in Carlsbad with a full lesson book. He's also a hell of a player with a zero handicap and competitive aspirations. It's another amazing golf comeback.

Silton's golf hero, Tiger, continued to play heroically after yet another round of surgery on his suspect knee, but then began his slow slide off Mount Olympus. Woods led the 2009 PGA Championship at Hazeltine with one round remaining, which is to say, he was certain to win the 2009 PGA Championship at Hazeltine. He had had *fifty* 54-hole leads or ties for the lead in his career and had won forty-seven of those tournaments. Playing the runner-up on Sunday would likely be a round-faced man from Seoul, whose Americanized name is Y. E. Yang.

Yang Yong-eun, thirty-seven, the son of a farmer of the volcanic soil on Jeju-do—the Hawaii of South Korea, its Honeymoon Island—had come late to golf. His world ranking at the start of the year had been 460, but he'd taken the Honda Classic in the spring—"from out of nowhere," as they say— and now his rank was nearly down to double digits. The world's number one golfer had won seventy professional tournaments by that point. Yang had won just the one.

That Saturday night, someone asked the world's 110th-ranked player what he thought the odds were of him winning.

"About seventy to one," he said.

Several accounts of the day allege that Tiger and Stevie attempted to discommode YY by never saying a word to him, by invading his space by standing too close, and by playing very slowly when it might ratchet up the pressure. If they did all that, it was out of character, and it didn't work.

When Y-Squared chipped in for eagle on fourteen, a short par four, he took a one-shot lead. On fifteen, he said to his caddie, "Tiger nervous."

Later, someone asked the South Korean man why *he* wasn't nervous. "It's not like you're in an octagon where you're fighting against Tiger and he's going to bite you or swing at you with his nine iron. The worst that I could do was just lose to Tiger," the wry Yang Yong-eun said. And then he told the lie all underdogs tell.

"So I really had nothing much at stake."

Nothing to lose, nothing at stake! Hilarious!

With a thrilling birdie on the final hole—remember that hybrid from 210 over the tree and over a bunker to a tight pin on eighteen?—the heretofore unknown Y. E. Yang beat Tiger Damn Woods seventy to seventy-five for the day and had won the PGA by three strokes. It was closer than that; Tiger bogied the final two holes in desperate attempts to make birdie. Nevertheless, the seventy-five was two shots higher than any round Tiger had ever had in winning his fourteen majors. He averaged 69.5 over those fourteen final rounds.

It looked so odd, so improbable, to see the other guy pumping his fist on the eighteenth green.

Three months later came a far worse setback.

• • •

Tiger had this reckless third life, as you know, and it ate up the other two.

I find that I have no taste for recounting the twists and turns in the Revelations of Sexual Misconduct. Besides, other outlets, such as contemporaneous issues of the *National Enquirer*, provide a far more thorough and enthusiastic re-telling than I could ever accomplish. I read a few of the stories and admit that I became smitten by the scandal sheet's punchy prose style, its clever use of the caps lock key, and the insertion of envy-making hot button words (the following example has two or three; see if you can spot them):

> **"BUT an ENQUIRER reporter in Melbourne watched as Rachel checked into the posh Crown Towers Hotel, and went up to the 35th floor, which houses the hotel's ritzy VIP Suite . . ."**
> **—this from NATIONAL ENQUIRER'S WORLD EXCLUSIVE of November 28, 2009**

But was anything believable in this cartoon of a newspaper? I know I want to read stories with headlines like "Mel Gibson: My Life as a Rabbit," "Al Gore's Diet is Making Him Stupid," and "Dying Man's Last Words Are Winning Lottery Numbers," but I won't believe the rabbit thing until Mel tells me about it himself.

The veracity of its reporting notwithstanding, the *National Enquirer* had real power and influence, and a substantial budget to fund its small army of informants (as you probably know, paying sources is strictly taboo in legitimate media). For example, the *Enquirer's* mercenary tattletales had snuffed the presidential campaigns of Democratic up-and-comers Gary Hart and John Edwards—an affair and a child out of wedlock—and besmirched the reputation of Rev. Jesse Jackson, by proving the existence of his "love child." Sex, murder (thank you, thank you, OJ), the British royal family, and miscellaneous celebrity disasters are the grist for its mill. The tabloid's tsk-tsk sex stories are written with an oddly Puritanical slant.

Who are its readers? Our readers are losers, the chief executive of the parent company said in 2017, in almost those words. "These are people that live their life failing so they want to read negative things about people who have gone up and then come down," David Pecker said in an interview with the *New Yorker*, apparently confident that his readers were unlikely to stumble across his casual slur. Pecker, as you will recall, was a key player in the Donald Trump/Stormy Daniels imbroglio.

Tiger had been on *National Enquirer's* radar since 2007. It was their usual thing: a tipster dropped a dime (in this case, the girl's mother); their operatives surveilled; then, bingo, the subject was observed canoodling in his Escalade with someone not named Elin. A "catch and kill" was, apparently, negotiated. In return for the *Enquirer's* agreement to not run "sin-sational!" words and photos, Tiger agreed to a cover story for its sister publication, *Men's Fitness,* in which he revealed the specifics of his heretofore secret workout routine.

Something similar occurred two years later with the above-mentioned Rachel. "She's dating Tiger," someone whispered to someone at the supermarket tabloid, and soon sharp-eyed people were following her, even to Melbourne, where the Australian Masters was being played, and in which Tiger was playing. Keteyian and Benedict lay it all out in *Tiger Woods,* as they had to, to produce a complete biography. I didn't, but prurient readers may enjoy Chapters 28 and 29. As Abraham Lincoln said—referring, I think, to something written by Walt Whitman, perhaps, *Leaves of Grass*: "People who like this sort of thing will find this the sort of thing they like."

You know the basic story. On Thanksgiving night, Elin, her suspicions aroused by the Rachel/Australia story in the *Enquirer,* searched her sleeping husband's cell phone for evidence, and found it. So mad she could hardly stand it, she awoke her mate, and a confrontation ensued. It was two in the morning. Tiger's mom was visiting . . . Fleeing Elin, he wrecked his black SUV. For reasons that remain in dispute, Mrs. Woods smashed both of the car's rear windows with a nine iron. Was it enough club?

I visited the crash site much later. Teams of uniformed landscapers clipped and primped the beautiful lawns of Isleworth that cool, clear winter morning and the drone of leaf blowers filled the air. I was impressed by how lovely and large the houses were, and by how fast the big Caddy must have been going to sideswipe a fire hydrant and to T-bone a tree, a sturdy live oak.

It's been a decade now and everyone's over it, but back then—well. The results were cataclysmic.

Within two weeks, thirteen more mistresses had come out, one or more of who had been paid to keep their big mouths shut. It was a perfect storm for the *Enquirer*—and for the non-celebrity-scandal based media, to be sure—because it was such a slow rolling disaster, like a serial, with new ex-lovers from the food and beverage industry and party girls and "actresses" emerging as Tiger inamorata day after day.

Sponsors dropped Tiger as if he were radioactive, and hot, and smelled bad. Accenture, the Ireland-based technology consulting company, said *slán*. AT&T bid Tiger adieu. Gatorade and Gillette terminated their deals. The thing with *Golf Digest* also ended, but that partnership had been winding down since before the Revelations. Procter & Gamble and Swiss watchmaker Tag Heuer backed away from their endorser while not actually ending the relationship. Only two of his big deals stayed intact, the ones with Nike and with EA Sports, the company that produced the wildly popular *Tiger Woods PGA Tour* video game.

Two weeks into the firestorm, the universe decreed that Tiger did not yet have enough to deal with. News emerged of an investigation into the practice of one Tony Galea, a Canadian sports medicine specialist who had paid a visit to the Woods house in Orlando. An alphabet soup of agencies—RCMP, FBI, ICE, DEA, as well as Homeland Security—was or soon would be examining exactly what Galea had in his needles and vials. Was that human growth hormone? Steroids? Those are illegal! Galea had had great success helping high-profile athletes recover from injury, among them Tiger and his friend Alex Rodriguez, the fabulous A-Rod.

With the *Enquirer* splashing big, red numbers on its front page as shorthand for the mistress count—9! for example—Big Humor rumbled to life. "Let's see what else is in the news. Oh! Another mistress came out today—how many is that now, Paul?"—late night monologists couldn't not include a Tiger reference. *Saturday Night Live* parodied CNN, with Jason Sudeikis as a mumbling Wolf Blitzer, and Kenan Thompson as Tiger wearing a golf club wrapped around his head and a tire track across his chest, apologizing to faux-Elin (Blake Lively) for running himself over with the car. On another *SNL* on another Saturday night, "Mistress #15" (Nasim Pedrad) is confused about a photograph of the other Tiger paramours. "I just thought they were me in different outfits and hairs," she said, a joke on how they looked so alike: blonde, mostly. Some of the vixens might have been valedictorians, but the funnier assumption was that they were all a little stupid.

In his "Doonesbury" comic strip, Garry Trudeau did a series in which the Tiger women decide that there are enough of them to form a union.

One of the most popular and successful athletes in history had become a joke. There are more painful things than getting publicly shamed and laughed at, but there aren't many.

The Tiger joke took a long time to tell. Pent-up envy, piling on, a touch of racism, and a widespread just desserts attitude gave it staying power. Besides, persistent public cruelty is OK in our great country as long as sex is involved. Murderers have an easier time. For example: How often did Jay Leno humiliate Monica Lewinsky on national television? Was there ever any recognition by Jay and his writers that there was a person in there?

But these were no laughing matters for Tiger. Before Christmas, Elin moved out, to an unfurnished house nearby, and she of course took the two kids with her. All four were together on Christmas day, and then Elin and the children were off for Sweden, to her twin sister and soulmate, to her home and family. I assume the unhappy couple suffered the soul-sick feeling of not being together for New Year's Eve and wondered if they ever would be again.

From late December to February 2010, Tiger did forty-five days in a sex addiction clinic in Hattiesburg, Mississippi. Some thought his Team was merely cynically medicalizing the problem to give Tiger some cover but the sheer number of extra-marital partners and the reckless disregard of his own and others' well-being argues otherwise. He was ill.

The Team hired former White House press secretary Ari

Fleischer to manage the crisis. Steinie strongly resisted the idea but Ari prevailed: apologize, he advised, as completely and as publicly as possible.

On February 19, an obviously repentant Tiger delivered a speech in a conference room at PGA tour headquarters in Florida. It was a stop the presses and turn on the TV moment. The keynote speaker would have to talk about his sex life with his mother in the front row and cameras on, a punishment straight from hell.

"I am deeply sorry for my irresponsible and selfish behavior I engaged in," he said.

"I have let you down. I have let down my fans.

"I brought this shame on myself.

"I have *never* taken performance-enhancing drugs.

"It's not what you achieve in life that matters, it's what you overcome."

His marriage? Still up in the air. He was not going to talk about it.

After about fourteen minutes of somber mea culpa, Tiger hugged his mother, Steinie, and longtime friend and Stanford golf teammate Notah Begay III. He then shook the hand of PGA tour commissioner Tim Finchem, who did not rise to his feet.

Stevie watched from the other side of the world, from his home in New Zealand. "Peculiar," he said about it later. "He was so awkward in his delivery and choice of words. Heavily scripted with nothing natural about it . . . I'm positive it was not his idea. It was obvious to those who knew him that it was not something he would do."

The big surprise for some Tiger watchers was his invocation, near the end, of religion. "Part of following this path [of recovery] for me, is Buddhism," he said. "People probably don't realize that I was raised a Buddhist and I actively practiced my faith since childhood until I drifted away from it in recent years."

People didn't realize it because Tiger had kept his religiosity a secret until that moment but this, we suppose, was the time to bring it up. In the surprisingly churchy (and Christian) Twelve Steps Program that many treatment programs embrace—including the one Tiger had just completed—steps two, three, five, six, seven, and eleven concern the addict reaching out to God, recognizing that only the help of God can see you through, that you are powerless without God, and so on.

But Buddhists seek to evolve and improve as *individuals* as they seek enlightenment. Buddhists don't believe in a savior or worship a god. Patient Woods would have to make do with only Six Steps.

• • •

Other athletes endured sex scandals. Baseball players Wade Boggs and Pete Rose, for example, also suffered from sex addiction, but as big as those marvelously efficient singles hitters were, they were nowhere close to defining their sport, as Tiger did his, and were not in his league in ten other ways, including popularity, influence, and income.

Had there ever been such a situation before? Who else in American sports and entertainment history occupied a perch as high as Tiger's and was brought down by indiscretion, and then got pummeled by a gleeful, leering press?

While not exactly analogous situations, perhaps O.J. Simpson (double murder)? Lance Armstrong (doping)? Mike Tyson (rape)? Michael Vick (animal cruelty)? Ray Rice (domestic abuse)? NBA superstar Kobe Bryant was publicly vilified for his infidelity as well (and nearly stood trial for rape), though his wife, Vanessa, took him back and he has since managed to rehabilitate his public image (and win an Oscar).

More recently there have been the Hollywood figures who have been brought down, deservedly so, by the "me too" movement, like Harvey Weinstein, Mario Batali, Kevin Spacey, and, perhaps most notably, Louis C.K. Yet with the exception of O.J.—who likely *murdered two people*—none of these cases elicited the kind of salacious public intrigue that Tiger's did. To find a true comparison—at least in terms of media frenzy—you'd, you'd have to go back about a hundred years, when a man from Kansas named Roscoe Arbuckle suffered a similar fate.

Little Roscoe got off to a bad start in life because he was not ever really little; although both his parents were slim, slight individuals, Baby Arbuckle arrived weighing a hefty thirteen pounds. Because he despised U.S. Senator Roscoe Conkling (R-NY), who had a deserved national reputation as womanizer, and believing the child was not his, the nominal father gave the child a cruel name: "Roscoe Conkling Arbuckle" rebuked both the mother and the bouncing baby boy every minute of every day. When Mary Arbuckle died twelve years later, following the unhappy family's move to Santa Ana, in Southern California, William would no longer support this big kid who he did not like and had never claimed.

Whatever his genetic inheritance, Roscoe had talent as a singer, the strange and wonderful agility of some big people, and a desire to perform. He won a talent competition less for his great voice than for avoiding the hook by cartwheeling into the orchestra pit. The crowd roared with laughter.

Audiences roared again when they saw the moon-faced young man in *A Noise from the Deep*, a 1913 silent film in which Arbuckle, soon to be known by one of his characters' names, "Fatty," had a pie thrown in his face. It was Hollywood's first pie and first face. Fatty could pitch a pie, too, with either hand, and he was accurate from ten feet. He became part of Mack Sennett's slapstick comedy movie troupe, joining Charlie Chaplin, and he became a star, one of the biggest, with his fee for a day on the set skyrocketing from five bucks a day to a thousand, a fabulous sum back then. In '21, he signed a deal with Paramount Pictures Corporation to make twenty-two films for $3 million.

"He was Falstaffian in size, if not in subtlety," reported the *New York Times*. "His popularity was universal, especially with the children."

But on September 5, 1921, at a Labor Day party in Fatty's suite at the Saint Francis Hotel in San Francisco, a very pretty twenty-five-year-old woman named Virginia Rappe became ill, and four days later died, of peritonitis caused by a ruptured bladder. It seems likely that of the many glasses of Prohibition era liquor she drank during the celebration, some of it had been adulterated. Methanol and other poisonous additives were, in fact, common in bootleg booze.

"Fatty could not have caused her death," says Dr. Al Oppenheim, the internist who we mentioned earlier in connection with Tiger's junior golf career. "Most likely, her chronic cystitis exacerbated by bad alcohol burst her bladder and led to the peritonitis that killed her."

Although the "evidence" against him seems laughable today, and his main accuser was thoroughly discredited—and was, in fact, attempting to extort him—the blind ambition of San Francisco District Attorney Murray pushed the case forward. Roscoe C. Arbuckle was arrested on September 10 and charged with murder. The theory of the crime was that the three-hundred-pound actor had forced himself on the poor woman, and, basically, crushed her. They placed the big man in a little room—Cell Number 12 in the San Francisco Hall of Justice, which at least one newspaper referred to as a "death cell." At the end of eighteen days there, the grand jury indicted him for manslaughter.

Crazy to Marry, Fatty's latest film, which was playing in theaters all over the country, was summarily withdrawn.

The trials of Fatty Arbuckle (there were three of them, resulting in two hung juries and an acquittal) were heaven-sent spectacles for the *San Francisco Examiner* and the other scandal-baiting papers of the Hearst chain. "Sold us more newspapers than the sinking of the *Lusitania*," William Randolph Hearst was said to have said.

Few knew that Arbuckle would not allow certain defense testimony in the first two trials, even though it might have ended the foolishness quickly, in his favor. Fatty was so much the gentleman that he wanted to spare Miss Rappe's family from hearing who their daughter really was.

The acquittal in March '22—after five minutes of deliberation—came with an apology. But the damage had been done. "Then came long years of Fatty Arbuckle's trial before public opinion," wrote the *New York Times* on June 30, 1933, in his obit. "His efforts at rehabilitation were entirely unsuccessful."

Arbuckle died of a heart attack in 1933, in his sleep, at the age of forty-six.

• • •

Fatty was more sinned against than sinning, but the scandal ruined him. Tiger's outcome wouldn't be that simple, because like a lot of us in the blackjack game of life, he was playing three hands. He might go bust in his personal life and in endorsements and he'd never be a SEAL, but the golf ball didn't know what he did last night, or care, and no one was kicking him out of their tournaments because his presence guaranteed their success. Unlike Fatty, who was blackballed even after his acquittal, Woods could still do the thing that gave his life meaning. On the other hand, Tiger could not ask for another take; he did what he did in front of a live audience. Had he lost the fans? No performer on a stage or between yellow nylon ropes can thrive if the people are laughing in the wrong places.

After the Hiatus in Hattiesburg, Tiger went back to his happy place, the practice tee. Hank flew into Orlando and they began to prepare for the big annual event in East Georgia. He practiced the big sweeping hook he might use off the tee on thirteen and the cut driver he'd hit through the chute and up the hill on eighteen. The Masters would be Tiger's first tournament after the Unpleasantness. He'd be ready.

If the Masters would be ready for him was another story, partly because of the sanctimony of His Holiness William "Billy" Payne, the Chairman of the Augusta National Golf Club, who used the dubious moral authority of his office to rub Tiger's nose in the mud.

On the Sunday before tournament week, Tiger played nine holes, then marched to the rectory. He had an audience with Himself. He kissed the ring, took a knee, entered the confessional—something. There's no video. Rabbi Payne spoke later.

"It is simply not the degree of his conduct that is so egregious here," he said in his annual address to the media on the day before the tournament began. "It is the fact that he disappointed all of us, and more importantly, our kids and our grandkids. Our hero did not live up to the expectations of the role model we saw for our children."

"Our hero" had fractured his family and lost his self-respect and people were laughing at him, but he hadn't been through enough, apparently, to suit pious Billy. How did Tiger keep from slugging him?

"Is there a way forward? I hope so," said Imam Payne. "Yes, I think there is. But certainly, his future will never again be measured only by his performance against par; but measured by the sincerity of his efforts to change."

We wonder why Billy thought he needed to take a shot from on high at Tiger, and why he couldn't have just kept his mouth shut on this topic.

Can you imagine an official in any other sport fretting about one of its players' "sincerity"? "We'd like to see better sincerity from Steph Curry this season," is a sentence the NBA commissioner Adam Silver will never utter. Stealing—of bases and of signs—it's in the game of baseball. So is taunting of the opposition's batsmen, even in the littlest little baseball leagues. Soccer's legions of floppers proudly showcase deceit. Basketball coaches teach tricks to exaggerate contact in order to draw a charging call (yell when you fall, and be sure to slap the floor with both hands). Football players purposely hold and trip and clip but there is no sanction unless a zebra throws a flag. A running back sprinting down the sideline with the ball will never ever stop and explain, "I stepped out of bounds back at the thirty. Sorry, I guess the back judge didn't see it." NFL Commissioner Roger Goodell is not without his own sanctimony. Just think about his comments in the wake of the aforementioned Michael Vick and Ray Rice cases.

But golf's unique ethical culture demands self-policing, unless your name is Trump. Golfers forego countless opportunities to cheat, and we call penalties on ourselves for infractions no one else could ever see or know. Sportsmanship is held out as the highest ideal. That eighteenth green ceremony we do with the handshakes and the hats off gets to the essence pretty well. No real golfer wants this messed with. Tradition, sportsmanship, honor: Good things.

Tiger crashed the honor of the game into the dishonor in his real life. What did that mean? Anything?

"The game's conceit is that it or The First Tee teaches you how to behave," observes golf industry executive John Strawn, author of *Driving the Green*. "So what happens when golf's greatest player is revealed to be a cheat and a liar? That's why the pushback was so strong from Billy Payne and others. Tiger's indiscretions threatened everything they believe in."

At last the wounded warrior enters the arena for practice rounds. Augusta and Augusta National are boiling with people; it's as crazy as '97 again, and media interest is through the roof. What hits the man has taken, we patrons think, hard hooks and haymakers to the chest, head, and ego. But Tiger proceeds with dignity, does the best he can in an impossible situation.

He has a game with the most laid-back guy around, Fred Couples, who is cared for by his equally low-key caddie, Joe LaCava. Tiger, hiding a bit, debuts a new look: wraparound shades.

Tiger's unusual ability to focus despite any distraction is vital now. He pulls his game face out of his locker and puts it on. He places focus, calmness, clarity—maybe a little kale—into a blender and drinks it down. With his Apology, he's manned up more than Bill Clinton ever did. He will play with his usual pride and flair because here the people love him and what's more, they *get* him. Connoisseurs of the golfing arts, Augusta National fans appreciate true genius.

The tune-a-mint begins.

What? You don't remember if Tiger won or lost the 2010 Masters? He lost! Big time. It was the worst tournament anyone ever had. He lost his wife, his instructor, his caddie, and the Masters.

In reverse order: Tiger didn't really "lose" the 2010 Masters. In fact, he played great, finishing in a tie for fourth, five shots back of the winner, Phil Mickelson. It was an amazing performance for a man who hadn't competed in four months.

But the relationship with Caddie Williams had deteriorated—a lot—since the big, bad story broke. Stevie had not been complicit in Tiger's extra-marital affairs but most everyone assumed he had been. Fed up with the haranguing press and with being *booed* after he'd won a car race at Bay Park in the North Island city of Tauranga, the New Zealander had repeatedly asked the Team for a statement clearing him of any involvement in the mess. No can do, they told him. Absolving you would shine a bad light on others in the entourage.

Stevie got some things off his chest before picking up the Nike bag again. In the car on the drive to the Orlando airport, from which they'd fly in Tiger's Gulfstream to Bush Field in Augusta, he made clear how furious he was to be dragged through a scandal he'd had nothing to do with, how awful it had made his and his family's life, that his calls had not been returned, and how the Team's indifference to his plight only ratcheted up his anger. Oh, and Tiger? another thing: you're not going to spit at the hole when you miss a putt anymore. And you're not going to just toss your club in the direction of the golf bag when you're through with it, making your caddie pick up the sticks off the ground, treating him as the lowest kind of servant instead of a partner.

Stevie wanted an apology, more respect, and better communication. Also, a raise.

The important subtext was that Williams didn't believe this sex addiction shit, not for a minute. To him, Tiger had simply been a pig who thought he could get away with it. Stevie and his wife were quite fond of Elin; as for Tiger, lately, not so much.

"I didn't have any sympathy over what he'd done," wrote Williams in his book. "I believe you're in charge of your own action and I have no sympathy for people who get addicted to drugs or gambling or sex. People make choices and he'd chosen to do this.

"But I did have sympathy for the way he had to suffer in front of the world when others would have been able to sort out their mess in private."

The bitter way their relationship was about to end flavors Williams's recollections. He does not recall a brave competitor facing the music but rather a sadly diminished former hero whose uppance had come.

"I could sense immediately that the air around us had changed," Williams wrote. "The attitude toward Tiger, usually deferential and distanced, was replaced by cool disdain. People all over the world, including his rivals, had lost their respect for him and were no longer in awe of him—his lies and double life had been exposed. He was naked out there."

A banner-pulling prop plane flew slowly over the course as Woods teed off to begin the first round. The sign read: TIGER: DID YOU MEAN BOOTYISM?

But the mood and the vibe improved. Other than the banner, the build-up and the first two rounds went great, from Stevie's point of view. Tiger seemed more humble and appreciative and it felt like a breath of very fresh air. But after Tiger met the press following his wonderful first two rounds—sixty-eight and seventy—Williams was shocked to hear Steinie tell Tiger that in order to win, he had to "stop being a nice guy" and go back being to his mean old self. Williams was shocked.

"[After] he had made a public commitment to a less snarling and aggressive Tiger, that he'd promised me to reform his bad habits, his main advisor was telling him the opposite," Williams would write. "Right then, something inside me changed . . . My immediate thought was 'I'm not going to be around much longer.'"

And yet: should we even give a damn about this caddie's work environment? At least two things say that we shouldn't. First, Stevie had been making about a million dollars a year for a dozen years. Second, Tiger Woods was no anonymous golf pro. Allowances were made for Beethoven, for Einstein, for Degas, for Ali. Was this genius less deserving? OK, he wasn't a people person on the golf course and he'd never be asked to sell time shares off it. He did some other stuff to make up for it.

A day and a half after Steinie told Tiger to get mean, another Team member felt the world turn. "It suddenly hit me," Haney wrote. "A very strong feeling that this would be the last time I ever worked for Tiger Woods."

Past slights and missed opportunities to say "thanks" had by then accumulated like old newspapers, and in the highly charged atmosphere of the first tournament back after the Revelations, everything seemed bigger, louder, more important. A new load of straw dropped on the camel's back.

Haney hated some of the things Tiger said in the Saturday night presser. "I don't have control of the ball," he observed, adding that he was suffering from a "two-way miss" (his ball could fly unpredictably right or left), which is poison for any golfer with the ambition to play well. Hank understood the comments as direct shots at himself, the sub-contractor for Tiger's swing.

Incredibly, despite every possible threat to his concentration short of a hostage situation, Tiger stood only four shots out of the lead after 54 holes. The man's competitiveness and laser beam focus knew no peer.

The potential of the final round didn't cheer him, however. Haney, facing a crabby student, tried and failed to say the right things during the pre-game on the range. At last, as Tiger left the practice green for the first tee, Hank tried "good luck." It would be their final words as a couple.

Tiger had a crazy up and down round that included a second shot hole-out on seven; it added up to sixty-nine, which was very good but not good enough. Mickelson won. Peter Kostis of CBS-TV steered the mic to Tiger's mouth. Here was the rare time when dipping a bucket into his deep well of clichés would be a good thing. Like, how wonderful it was to be back and how amazing the fan support had been and how about this great weather. Instead the unhappy warrior was churlish and caviled again about his swing. Haney resigned that night, in a phone call to Steinie.

In their books, neither Haney nor Williams mention one

obvious factor in their client's bad mood. Didn't they sub-scribe to the *National Enquirer*'s website? For on Wednesday, the day before the Masters began, *NE* broke another mistress story, only this one wasn't like the others. The woman involved was the daughter of a neighbor, a twenty-one-year-old college girl the Woodses had known since she was fourteen. Tiger had owned up to many flings, including dalliances with adult performers, but not to this one. It seemed to be the last straw. Elin filed. She got custody of the children and about $100 million.

• • •

And so began Tiger's decade in the wilderness.

His personal life doesn't lend itself to data points—whose does?—but golf results are basically math, after all, and his plainly traced a bell curve. In October 2010, after five-plus years at the top, he lost his world #1 ranking, to Lee Westwood. With his health and swing deteriorating, he played only nine events in 2011 and saw his ranking fall to 52. The Tiger trajectory swooped dramatically up when he won three times in 2012 and five more times in '13—career totals for a very good Tour player—but thereafter, the abscissa and the ordinate on his graph showed only bad news. He was getting older. He was accomplishing less. His world ranking in 2015 slipped to 254.

Following Hank's resignation at the end of that awful week in Augusta, Team Tiger had an important slot to fill. A couple of months later, a *GQ*-looking chap named Sean

Foley auditioned for the job at the Team's rental house at the PGA Championship at Whistling Straits in Wisconsin. Hard to say now if it was a very tough or a very receptive crowd, for Tiger had just shot eighteen over in the previous tournament, the Bridgestone Invitational, at Firestone, an event he had won seven times. At any rate, Foley got the job.

"Sean was super-convincing," Stevie recalled. "Even if his language was incomprehensible"—neural pathways and fascial chains and so on. On the other hand, one of Foley's main messages was easy enough to grasp. *Lean into it, big guy*, he told the boss. You're falling back too much.

A Canadian who lived and taught golf in Orlando, Foley was Tiger's age, roughly—both were in their mid-thirties. Perhaps a fellow Gen Xer would be good to work with. Hank was Tiger's senior by twenty years and Butch was thirty-two years older than his number one student. Besides, Haney and Harmon weren't only old, they were old school, their baseline thinking about golf instruction having been informed by a book, *Five Lessons*, that had been published in 1957.

Sean Foley was a kettle of fish of a different color.

First of all, he spoke biomechanics, not Hogan catchphrases. He used video and Doppler radar-based TrackMan during his lessons. He listened to rap music. His father is a Scot, his mother a West Indian from Guyana. Although he didn't look the part, he'd attended and played golf at an historically black college, Tennessee State. Foley was often shunned at TSU—for lack of adequate pigment, presumably.

It made him tougher, he told Charles McGrath of the *New York Times:*

"So now when people ask me what it's like being Tiger's coach and all those terrible things people say, I'm like, whatever. It doesn't bother me at all."

2010 had ended with no wins for Tiger. Or for Williams, who considered them his, too. Since the Revelations and the Team's awkward handling of the aftermath vis-à-vis the caddie, the looper's relationship with the boss had devolved to business only. He was looking at the door. And he walked through it, or was pushed through it, the next summer.

Stevie had given Adam Scott an impromptu pep talk just before the final round of the '11 Masters, and the encouragement had spurred the tall Aussie to a sixty-seven, and almost a win. So when Tiger was hurt and not playing in the next major, the US Open, it was no big surprise that Scott called to ask if Williams could be his bearer for the week. He said yes, Tiger gave his permission, and it was done. Scott missed the cut.

Two weeks later, with Tiger still injured and unable to play, it was the same thing, only this time it was an argument. Stevie explained that this was merely another one-off, it wasn't him quitting. Tiger said OK, reluctantly. Later, he changed his mind. There were back-and-forths involving the player, the caddie, and Steinie.

The last conversation went like this, roughly:

If you caddie for Adam, we're finished.

Then we're done.

And another long relationship bit the dust. The bad blood of it became plain at the 2011 Bridgestone in Akron. Tiger, with Fred Couples's ex, Joe LaCava, on the sack, finished way down the list, and Scott won. Then, the oddest thing: David Feherty of CBS-TV stuck the mic under the caddie's nose. That *never* happens; Stevie wasn't ready—why would he be? He was too emotional, too caught up in the moment. "*This* is the greatest win of my career," he blurted out, although it wasn't even close.

In early March 2012, advance copies of *The Big Miss* hit the street and Steinie's ire hit code red, but he should have been mad at himself for forgetting to have Hank sign a non-disclosure agreement. The revelations about Tiger's SEAL obsessions—and the popsicle—caused the most comment.

Meanwhile, Foley's high-tech coaching was working. Although uncharacteristically bad weekend rounds kept Tiger far away from the trophy in three of the majors, and his 0-3-1 record in the Ryder Cup did not impress (Europe won)—there were very bright spots, too. He took the Arnold Palmer Invitational for his first win in two years. By winning two other tournaments, including Nicklaus's event, the Memorial, the Marvelous Mr. Woods passed Jack in career wins with seventy-four. Another result had to be encouraging, a tie for third in the Open Championship at Royal Lytham, four shots back of the new Champion Golfer of the Year, Ernest Els.

And he met a girl. Not just any girl. She was a spectacular,

Amazonian individual, a taller, more muscular Elin. She was Ms. Vonn, the world champion skier, who had just been divorced from Mr. Vonn, also a skier.

Relationships require skillful give and take to work, as well as luck, magic, and some other element hidden to me, perhaps astrology. Lindsey and Tiger may have checked every box but they had a serious challenge few face: their great fame. They had little access to the sort of routine activities most of us can enjoy, such as bowling or dropping in on a whim at happy hour at Applebee's. Theirs was the low-oxygen altitude of high-profile dating that required an announcement when they started up and another when their thing fizzled two and a half years later.

They came out as a couple at the 2013 Masters, where an incident occurred that was, maybe, a referendum on the erstwhile hero. Haters would find a new reason to hate; supporters had to keep pointing out that Tiger not only wasn't trying to hide an infraction, he didn't bitch when he got a two shot-penalty on top of a one-shot penalty. A human hair away from an eagle three on fifteen, he wound up with an eight. It might have cost him the tournament.

You may remember it: in the second round, Tiger hit a perfect third shot on the fifteenth that became perfectly dreadful. So accurate was this wedge that the ball clanged into the bottom of the pin and bounced into the pond in front of the green. And the crowd groaned. Bummer!

Now what? Tiger had three options to get a ball back in

play, all of them costing a one-shot penalty: play from a spray-painted circle close to the pond; find the spot where the water ball made a ripple, line it up with the pin, then hit a ball along that vector from as far back as he wanted; or, play again from the original spot. Tiger took option three, but he did it wrong. Instead of playing from the original spot he backed up a few yards, dropped a new pelota from shoulder height, hit a beautiful shot, and holed the short putt for a bogey six. Which should have been an eight, with a two-shot penalty for the incorrect drop. Which made the scorecard he signed incorrect. Which requires disqualification. Which was not done, because the next morning Masters rules officials cited a new rule, 33-7, which allows penalties to be assessed after the fact, in "extraordinary circumstances."

Were these circumstances extraordinary enough? A brouhaha brewed almost to the point of drowning out the competition. Innocent mistake, wrote Thomas Boswell in the *Washington Post*, let's get on with it. Not so fast, said commentator Brandel Chamblee on The Golf Channel: "It's incumbent on him to disqualify himself. Anything else is frankly unacceptable."

Tiger went Boswell. Had he gone Chamblee, he'd have avoided the possibility of being helped into a green jacket with a little asterisk on the breast pocket. And it would have been a PR masterstroke for a guy who needed one. "Reasonable people have questioned the legitimacy of my score," he could have said. "I choose to withdraw to end the controversy. I will not put myself above the game."

Anyway—he played. Finished in a tie for fourth. Adam Scott won. As is the winning caddie's right, Stevie took the cloth off the stick on eighteen, adding to his collection of captured battle flags.

And then:

Achilles tendon, lumbar disc, wrist, elbow, neck, medial collateral ligament. Sciatica, muscle spasms, and shooting pain.

Repeat: Achilles tendon, lumbar disc, wrist, elbow, medial collateral ligament. Sciatica, muscle spasms, and shooting pain.

Tiger's aching body parts led to many withdrawals and DES's (Didn't Even Start) at the end of 2013 and beyond. Finally, it led to surgery on his spine, which may once have represented an I'm-just-going-to-watch-the-game-on-TV, permanent time out for an athlete but does not now. With the use of a wonderful instrument called an endoscope, the micro-discectomy for a surgeon is like an oil change for a car mechanic. Maybe a valve job is a better comparison: removing bone from the back to free up a nerve is very serious business, and a misstep could have terrible consequences.

But Tiger had wonderfully skilled surgeons, of course, and each of his various "procedures" was deemed a success, at least in post-op. He had his first micro-discectomy in March 2014; the second, in September 2015; and a third back surgery just a month later, to "relieve discomfort." His pain may have been alleviated—on some days, at least—but his golf . . .

In April 2016, someone asked Butch Harmon about his former student. "I don't know if Tiger can ever come back," he said. "God, I hope so. It would be so good for the game. But Tiger can't do mediocre."

But he did. He did mediocre and worse. It was as if some impostor had stepped into his shoes and put on his swooshes. Someone who looked like Tiger shot eighty-two in Phoenix and eighty-five at the Memorial; this same guy had the chip yips, golf's second most comical malady. Only chronic shanks induce more suppressed laughter. Unless you're the yipper or the shanker, of course, in which case you want to kill yourself.

On "The Dan Patrick Show" in August '18, MBE Sir Nick Faldo, thrice a Masters winner, revealed a sad comment from Tiger at the Masters Champions dinner from two years before. His three back surgeries had failed, Tiger said. "He whispered, 'I'm done, my back is done. I won't play golf again,'" said Nick. "He was in agony, he was in pain . . . He couldn't move."

With a desire to live a normal life as his stated purpose, Tiger tried a riskier, more invasive surgery in April 2017: spinal fusion. It's not an unusual operation; bad baby boomer backs are one big reason for the roughly 600,000 disc fusions performed in the US last year. Why do the 600,000 do it?

For pain relief. What do they get? Stability, at the cost of flexibility. As for the pain . . .

In a study quoted by Gina Kolata in the *New York Times*, about half of the people getting lumbar (lower) spine fusions used opioids to help manage the pain. Post-op, nine percent stopped with the Vicodin or whatever. But thirteen percent who had not used opioids before became long-term users.

Tiger was in the largest group, that used before and after.

"It's hard to know what constitutes success," Kolata wrote. "By [one] definition—more than thirty percent relief of pain and thirty percent improvement in function—only about half of fusion operations succeed."

In mid-April of 2017, Dr. Richard Guyer of the Center for Disc Replacement at the Texas Back Institute in Plano, Texas, performed Tiger's Anterior Lumbar Interbody Fusion. Dumbed down: Dr. Guyer removed the bottom disc in the patient's back and put in its place a metal cage packed with bone harvested either from a cadaver or from the patient's hip. Exact details were not forthcoming, given doctor-patient confidentiality. As usual, everyone declared the operation a success—in that no one died, we suppose. Whether the procedure had been worth the trouble wouldn't be known for months. Meanwhile, pain would be Tiger's constant companion.

About a month later it got to be too much. You may have heard: at two in the morning on May 29, 2017, officers from the Palm Beach County Sheriff's Department found Tiger asleep at the wheel by the side of the road fifteen miles from his home. The somnolent man was invited to step out of the vehicle. He was dressed in cargo shorts, a Nike t-shirt, and untied shoes. After earning an F in the field sobriety test, the cops cuffed him, which may be standard operating procedure but nevertheless seems ridiculous given the prisoner's condition. At the station they snapped a mug shot and then it was state your name and your height and weight and your hair and eye color and blow into this tube and sit over there and do you want a lawyer.

We don't have to guess how badly Tiger was feeling. The tox screen is eloquent on that score. He was in pain; he'd taken two drugs for that, Dilaudid (hydromorphone) and Vicodin (hydrocodone). His mood was cratering; two drugs for that, too, Xanax and THC, the psycho-active component in marijuana. And because he was sick from pain and anxiety or depression, he couldn't sleep, and so had swallowed Ambien.

Two opiates, two sedatives, and THC amounted to a very dangerous drug cocktail. Accidental overdose deaths are an epidemic in the US—an incredible and appalling 70,237 of them occurred in 2017—and are the leading cause of death for Americans under age fifty. Traffic deaths on American roads in '17 totaled a little over 40,000. If Tiger had died by crashing his Mercedes that night, someone would have to decide which category he belonged in.

"I feel like [it was] a massive scream for help," said

Michael Phelps, the swimmer, who'd been treated for addiction. He befriended Tiger.

The next day's often used headline—DUI of the Tiger— was clever but not that funny. Because most of us have been affected directly or indirectly by an overdose death. And most of us recognized a man hitting bottom, because we've been there, or almost there, ourselves.

• • •

Hogan, Silton, Alexander, Peete, and Sifford were run over by a bus, shot through the head, burned to toast in a plane crash, deprived, deformed, and rejected—respectively. These golfers achieved great things despite the barriers placed in their way by capricious fortune and their stories inspire us. For contrast, we looked briefly at Arbuckle, who suffered but did not endure.

But before we hum "Eye of the Tiger" and imagine a movie montage of sweat, pain, and sacrifice leading to Tiger's epic return to the mountaintop, let's look at one last comeback story. Maybe hers was the greatest of them all.

It's difficult today to overstate the celebrity of Mildred Ella "Babe" Didrikson Zaharias. The lantern-jawed daughter of Norwegian immigrants was as big as Tiger, and was to women's sports what Secretariat would become to horse racing. Like Tiger, she grabbed the world's attention as a teenager, when she was the best player on the best basketball team in the land. She threw a baseball three hundred feet in the air. She won the sewing competition in the South

Texas State Fair. She won the 1932 AAU national track and field championship—by herself. No teammates are needed when you enter eight events, win five, and tie for first in a sixth. A month later, in the Olympics in Los Angeles, she set three world records in three disparate events—80-meter hurdles, high jump, and javelin. Two golds and a silver, on a technicality.

Babe was therefore the anti-Tiger in a way, a generalist of a genius who could do a lot of things exceptionally well. Tiger had been a specialist since he was in diapers and never deviated into quoits or quilting or anything else, until he discovered the undersea world as a diver in 2003.

After the Olympics, the twenty-one-year-old greatest woman athlete on earth played eighteen holes for the first time and shot about 100. But she liked it. Three years later she dominated her new game, winning fourteen amateur tournaments in a row at one point. Miss Didrikson could even beat boys. She qualified—she was not invited—for four PGA tour events and made the thirty-six-hole cut in three of them. Annika Sorenstam played pretty well at The Colonial in 2003, but her 145 didn't get her to the weekend. Babe's the only woman to have made a cut in the U.S. men's league (Michelle Wie once made a cut in a men's tournament in Asia, in the SK Telecom Open).

The one cut of the four the Babe didn't make came at the 1938 Los Angeles Open, when she was paired with and distracted by a friendly bear of man, a professional wrestler and kindred spirit named George Zaharias. They were married within the year. Big George—who played a bad guy in wrestling's jock opera—needlessly inflated his wife's accomplishments when there were notebooks out, and Babe played along.

Oh, the minds she blew. She didn't have any trace of the shyness gene. She had more ham in her than a prize pig. Biographer Don Van Natta tells the tale beautifully in his book, *Wonder Girl.*

In 1950, with a double handful of other women, she founded the LPGA. Everyone knew who the star was. Fellow pro Shirley Spork remembered her friend walking up to any group in the locker room or on the practice tee and saying, "Well, the Babe's here. Who's going to be second? Maybe you, Louise?"

Louise Suggs—one of the greatest woman golfers ever— hated Babe. Hated her. Others in and around the game complained that the Babe's muscled shoulders were too square, her walk and her manner were too masculine, and that although she was married to Mr. Zaharias, she was sleeping with Miss Dodd, meaning fellow LPGAer Betty Dodd. Babe didn't just break the rules of athletic femininity, she ground them under her heel and said, screw you. Once, in front of a big crowd, when it got too warm, she simply wiggled out of her half-slip. Shocking!

She wasn't exactly Ms. Sportsmanship, either. "I don't think I've ever seen anyone take losing less gracefully," said

Betsy Rawls of her old friend and rival. But the fans adored her as much as they would Arnie and, later, Tiger.

Colon cancer struck in 1953. The disease was much more frequently fatal then than now, and was practically a taboo subject, besides. But if Babe despaired, she did so in private. She used her platform to tell people to, for heaven's sake, get tested, and thereby surely saved some lives.

She had an -ectomy and an -ostomy. The press covered her recovery in the same breathless way as four years before, when America's Patient was named Hogan: "BABE WALKS, EATS SOLID FOOD" and "BABE TAKES RIDE, NOW FEELS BETTER" were typical all-caps headlines.

Her energy began to wane, but no way would she just stay at home with George and die. Four months after her cancer surgery, she teed it up in Chicago and finished third.

Ed Sullivan's people called. Would the Babe come on the show? Back in the day when your TV broadcast only three or four channels, watching Ed Sullivan's Sunday night variety show was a national ritual. Yes, Babe would be happy to appear. But she would not just appear; she would perform. So after the cadaverous host introduced his athletic guest, said guest said, "Thanks for all the cards and letters" and then produced her M. Hohner Marine Band Model #1896 harmonica and blew out a peppy version of "Begin the Beguine" in the key of C, complete with wah-wah and tremolo effects produced with her right hand. Ed asked for an encore. Babe's protege, Miss Betty Dodd, came up on the stage with her guitar and they played "Little Train A-Chuggin'."

From New York, the golfers/musicians went to Chicago and cut a record for Mercury (A-side: "I Felt a Little Teardrop". B-side: "Detour"). "BABE EMBARKS ON HILL-BILLY MUSIC CAREER" reported United Press International the next day.

Babe played two tournaments early in '54, and won them both, but she was like a clock running down. That summer, she traveled to Boston for the Big One. With major nursing help from Betty, Mrs. Zaharias sprinted to a big lead at Salem Country Club after two rounds. But US Opens for men and for women required a thirty-six-hole finale. Sound familiar? Was she up to the standard of Skip Alexander and Ben Hogan?

Well . . .

Hell, yes! Babe bogied a bunch of holes at the end, but she finished. And she won—by twelve. When her putt from eighteen feet to win by thirteen *just* missed, she did a little shimmy, and her adoring gallery stood and cheered. She had to be exhausted, but she wouldn't show it.

"Just eighteen months after a cancer operation," said the big voiced man on the newsreel. "Here she is, winning by a mile. One of the most inspiring comebacks in sports history!"

Cancer returned to Mrs. Zaharias soon after the '54 US Open, if it had ever left. She wasted away. Over a period of more than a year and a half when she was largely bedridden,

Betty Dodd and her guitar were the Babe's constant companions. "Ninety percent of the time she was in the hospital, George wasn't there. He didn't want to fool with it," Betty told me in 1990. "I used to play for her. Ballads, mostly. I didn't necessarily *want* to play."

Near the end, surgeons severed her spine in an effort to alleviate the pain. On what everyone knew would be her final Christmas with her dear friends, the Bowens, in Fort Worth, Babe said, I just want to see a golf course one last time.

The Bowens' yacht-like Cadillac rolled through a side gate at Colonial Country Club and stopped on a maintenance road. Babe got out of the car and hobbled up a slight rise to the second green. She knelt. For a few long moments the dying star ran her hands back and forth over the grass.

PART THREE

Fire At It

—

"All great events hang by a hair. The man of ability takes advantage of everything and neglects nothing that can give him a chance of success; whilst the less able man sometimes loses everything by neglecting a single one of those chances."

—Napoleon

Sunday, April 7

"Almost miraculous."

The words of the week are always "usually" and "always." As in "I always eat at Rae's Coastal Cafe on Tuesday night and I usually have the shrimp pâté and jerk chicken" or "they always put the pin front left on number six on Sunday" or "we usually rent the same house at Jones Creek every year" and "we always get drunk on Jameson whiskey at the Irish Tourist Irish Board party." Rituals are a crucial part of the fun at the only one of golf's four majors to return to the same place year after year.

Masters rituals make people happy. Happy people have one more drink than when they're at home. They order bigger steaks, tell better jokes, and make better friends—and all that sweet stuff becomes part of the ritual, too.

My same-as-always pattern requires a Tuesday arrival to gear up for the big Wednesday game in Waynesboro, a little town down in Burke County that bills itself as The Bird Dog Capital of the World. Waynesboro Country Club is no dog, however, and it takes great pride in not gouging your eyes out during Masters Week, unlike virtually every other golf course and hotel in the Central Savannah River Area. Twenty-five bucks for eighteen holes and a cart. Beer is just a dollar and a half per can, and it is cold. Better give me ten.

First among the communicants in Waynesboro is Tat Thompson, a retired Augusta banker, and an animated and masterful first tee debater. On this special day, he paces the grassy stage like an electrified Baptist preacher on a hot Sunday morning. "No, no, no, that's not gonna work!" says Tat. His Georgia accent is thick enough to slice and put on bread. "I want Mully, Danny, and Tim. Ten dollahs a man. Non holes. Four-man Lauderdale. What do you say, Baggah?"

For reasons unknown, I am "Bagger Vance" to Tat, whose overmatched opponents in the negotiations are Danny Fitzgerald, Tim Wright, the Ash and Hopkins brothers, Mike Rucker, Doc Coleman, Brian Leonard, Walt the Pharmacist, and several other colorful and budget conscious personalities. Sometimes—depending on degree of drunkenness—we retire to Tat's house to convene an après golf game of Termite, which is three-card guts.

"A tradition unlike any other," Jim Nantz says, but he could drop the A and add an s to convey a truer sense of the place. It's all of a piece: from the glory game at Waynesboro to the flabby egg salad and pimiento cheese sandwiches you always buy at the concession stand to the right of thirteen to the holy of holies, the Champions Dinner on Tuesday night. In the chill of first light on Thursday morning, a couple of beloved old pros always get the thing started by whacking out a tee ball, and they always will. (And don't you love how hard Gary Player grinds away at his only shot of the day?)

TV, too. For those of us—which is most of us—who watch from the couch, it's vitally important to hear the same CBS voices year after year. The sixteenth hole is just a short shot over a shallow pond unless there is sonorous commentary from Henry Longhurst, or his successor, Ben Wright, and now Verne Lundquist. Pat Summerall moderated the show from 1968 until Nantz took the helm twenty years later. Both were/are superb, but two anchors in fifty years? That's quite enough change, thank you.

What with having played in twenty-one of them, Tiger undoubtedly has his own Masters rituals, including winning (four times) or almost winning (top tens nine other times).

He usually arrives on Monday of tournament week but Caddie LaCava convinced the boss to get to town a day early this year, for a bit of extra time to acclimate to the speed of the greens.

It was a quick trip. Tiger's sexy sixteen-passenger Gulfstream G550 traversed the five hundred-odd miles from Palm Beach to Augusta Regional Airport in about an hour. Adam Scott, owner of the same model rocket ship, parked his at Daniel Field, Augusta's close-in private strip. Within days, the little airport would be a jam-packed parking lot for hundreds of millions of dollars-worth of corporate jets. The G550 alone sets you back about $42 million.

With the two Woods kids, new girlfriend Ms. Erica Herman, the family dog, and maybe some others ensconced at a beautiful riverside rental house in North Augusta, Tiger and Joey convened at the National. Which was crowded, what with the eighty youthful contestants in the Drive, Chip, Putt contest and their parents, friends, and fans. The Golf Channel covered the feel-good competition; stars included nine-year-old Angela Zhang of Bellevue, Washington, a seventy-five pounder who won her age group by clobbering a drive 189 yards. Former Masters champs—including the defender, Patrick Reed—handed out trophies and posed for photos. Other green jacket guys doing the grip and grin were Scott, Bubba Watson, Nick Faldo MBE, Mark O'Meara, Bernhard Langer, and Mike Weir.

But Woods wouldn't wait with the other winners; Woods would be working. And he had a secret.

"I told Joey I'd been grinding my butt off at home," Tiger recalled in a fascinating interview with Henni Zuel of GolfTV. "And I said, 'I'm not playing today, but I'll chip and putt.'"

So he did, on the first nine greens, and "just worked on speed" and the unusually large amount of break in Augusta National greens.

And presumably, during this interval, he told his looper about the secret he'd found in the dirt on the practice tee back in Florida: "a swing in which I could start drawing the ball. Because I don't have the length I used to have . . . I've lost a little bit off my fastball. So I've got to rely on my driver. And I found I could hit a draw with [every club] and [still] maintained the ability to hit a slider . . .

"And so I went like, OK, we got something here."

In layman's terms, Tiger had uncovered his latent ability to hit and control a right to left curveball, aka a draw. The draw and its annoying big brother, the hook, are good to have in your quiver at the left-bending holes at Augusta National, including but not limited to two, nine, ten, and thirteen. Furthermore, hooks and draws hit the ground running, making them a useful, if perilously aggressive technique for anyone pursuing greater distance off the tee. The "slider" Tiger referred to is a safety shot, a defensive left-to-right spinner that doesn't go as far as a draw but is usually easy to find. Also known as a fade.

That Tiger would be animated about ball flight did not seem to be in the cards when last we saw him, in May of '17, when he was groggy and disoriented and under arrest in the middle of the night at the Palm Beach County Sheriff's Department. But he did what he had to do after that.

Checked himself into a drug dependency clinic and graduated. Pled guilty to reckless driving. Handled his fifty hours of community service although I don't know how. Entered a DUI first-offender program and completed that, too.

As for the back. Well . . .

"It's almost miraculous," Jack Zigler, the president of the International Society for the Advancement of Spinal Surgery, told Adam Kilgore of the *Washington Post*. "On the one hand, you have somebody who's in great physical condition and extremely well motivated—it's the ideal patient. But on the other hand, he's going back to an unbelievable level of function. The likelihood you could ever get back there is small."

Credit belongs to the surgeon, to 21st-century medical technology, and to the patient. Given his appetite for hard work and workouts, Tiger did not have to fight the tendency of most back patients to move very slowly if at all. Instead he rehabbed like his golf career depended on it, which it did. He was a man with no Plan B and therefore very dangerous. Then, incredibly, he won the 2018 Tour Championship.

While Tiger and Joe skipped from green to green that sunny Sunday afternoon, another Nike-wearing early arriver, Brooks Koepka, slugged balls on the practice range.

Woods and Koepka had taken up residence in the same headline seven months earlier. At the 2018 PGA Championship at Bellerive, in St. Louis, they'd finished one-two, with Brooks as the one, and Tiger second by two.

They absolutely scorched the place; in the second round on the final green, Brooks hit the lip with a putt for a sixty-two, which would have been the lowest score ever shot in a major. Tiger's final round tee shots flitted about like a mosquito inside a car, but he made every putt and shot sixty-four.

"Woods, who in his youthful pomp was accustomed to obliterating courses and fields in the manner now the domain of Koepka, nodded in approval," wrote Ewan Murray in the *Guardian*.

"'He's driving it 330 yards in the middle of the fairway,' said [Tiger]. 'He's got nine irons for approach shots when most of us are hitting five irons or four irons, and he's putting well. That adds up to a pretty substantial lead.'"

Exactly. What with wins in the 2017 and 2018 US Opens, and now the '18 and '19 PGAs, might Brooks be the new Intimidator? Might the soon-to-be world number one frighten even Tiger? We've never seen that before. Here's Ewan Murray again, regarding Koepka's unusual unflappability: "The 28-year-old makes great play of the fact that golf does not excite him, which makes one wonder what on earth he would achieve if invigorated."

But no rivalry simmers between these Florida neighbors; there's no conscious psychological warfare. "Other than me and my team, everybody was rooting for Tiger—as they should," Koepka said from the winner's circle at Bellerive. "He's the greatest player ever to play the game and to have the comeback he's having is just incredible." Not exactly fightin' words.

No conscious psychological warfare . . . but who can doubt that Koepka scares the hell out of his peers with his physical presence and his play and his exploding stardom? He holds himself apart. At the AT&T Byron Nelson Invitational in May, a month after this Masters, Koepka arrived at the range on Wednesday amid a chevron of support staff: one caddie, two agents, and three other gentlemen who could have been an instructor, a physio, and a Nike rep (or maybe a cook; I know he has a cook). Although the Trinity Forest Golf Club practice tee is over a hundred yards wide and it wasn't particularly crowded, Team Koepka parked way off to the side, not even on the tee, and Brooks hit balls diagonally at the target greens in the center.

His practice session concluded, the broad-shouldered pro and his staff re-formed their armada and sailed toward the exit. My deadline loomed. It was time to be rude. I invaded their space. They quickened their pace. I introduced myself, asked Brooks for a chat at his convenience, and handed him a book, *The Masters*. Great for a sleepless night, I said, ha-ha.

"Thanks," he said, and handed the paperback to his agent as if it were a cents-off coupon for Shake 'n Bake. Which is to say, quickly.

"Not a reader, eh Brooks?" I said, giving up.

"I read!" he said, and then he was gone.

Monday, April 8

"His Ownself"

This was going to be a long week for Jerry Tarde and Michael O'Malley and the others in the *Golf Digest* house because of where they'd been and the thoughts they'd had a month before. That was when they flew from Kennedy or LaGuardia to DFW, rented cars, and found their way to a white stone cathedral in downtown Fort Worth. There they heard and delivered little speeches, looked blankly out into space, and listened to the walkout music at the end of the ceremony: "We'll Meet Again," an optimistic World War II anthem by a toothy English pop singer named Vera Lynn. Dan Jenkins chose the music. Jenkins, the heart and the funny bone of *Sports Illustrated, Golf Digest*, numerous novels, and the Thomas A. Edison of modern sports writing, died on March 7. He was ninety.

"I grew up reading Dan Jenkins," Editor-in-Chief Tarde told the congregation. "It shaped my life."

"I was Dan's editor. It was a twenty-three-year collaboration. It didn't feel like a job," said Executive Editor O'Malley when it was his turn. "He'd make you think and laugh at the same time."

Tarde and O'Malley and their writers and staffs would carry on because that's what you do but . . . the Masters without Jenkins? It wasn't going to be the same. It wasn't going to be as good. For not only did Dan turn in copy that made everyone proud, and tell a story that made everyone laugh, he was a holder of court, and an organizer of fun you never wanted to stop.

"There was something called the Jenkins Races," Tarde recalled. "At about 9:30 p.m., someone would bring in the next day's pairing sheets. There'd be seven or eight guys around a table. 'OK, low pair,' Dan would say, and we'd place our bets. Or high foreigner, low man, high pair. Dan was commissioner; he'd appoint a secretary to keep track of things. Frank Hannigan [a high priest of the USGA and yet a fun and funny man] would call in. Then we'd all forget who we'd bet on. It was one of the really great social events of the week."

For thirty years or so, Jenkins moderated another table in the library area on the second floor of the Augusta National clubhouse. A varying cast of golf and literary giants toasted the night and debated the great issues. I'd have wanted to be there any time when Bob Drum got wound up; as counterpoint to the eloquently profane golf writer for the *Pittsburgh Press,* I'd select the simply eloquent: Tom Brokaw, George Plimpton, Dave Marr, Ben Crenshaw, Herbert Warren Wind, Summerall, and Nantz. And Dan, of course. "Players are dumber today," he might say to get the ball rolling. Or "the LPGA needs shorter shorts."

Jenkins covered the Masters—in person, of course—sixty-eight times. He loved the event enough to criticize it, such as when its administrators were dumb enough to let the greens get soft. In fact, despite his pointed, mordant wit, he loved a lot of things about golf and golf tournaments and golfers, but he put only one man on a pedestal: his Fort Worth homeboy, Ben Hogan. Dan was Ben's tireless defender and advocate. "Ben Hogan worked harder, overcame more, and achieved more than just about any athlete you can name," Jenkins wrote in a blurb for my 1996 biography, *Hogan*. "I was privileged to cover many of his most thrilling victories, and I still place that among my most treasured memories of a lifetime of writing about sports."

As Hogan faded Dan became a confidante of Palmer. When Arnie's star dimmed Dan and Nicklaus became tight. Jack lost his luster and Tiger . . . wouldn't say a damn word. Although both Jenkins and Woods drew a paycheck from *Golf Digest*, Tiger refused every request for an interview with the Dean of American Sportswriters. It would have been easy; Jenkins was there for all fourteen of Tiger's major wins. For example: Hank Haney and Jenkins both stayed in the magazine's rental house during the 2006 Open Championship at Royal Liverpool. All week, after their post-round practice session, Tiger dropped his teacher off at the house, but refused invitations to come inside for a beer or a chat or a game of darts. He won that week, as you'll recall.

"We have nothing to gain" from a sit-down with Jenkins, Steinie said, short-term thinking that did not serve his client well, for we can think of a time when Tiger could have used an important friend in the media. Possibly the Team feared a give and take or a perjury trap with the quick-witted writer. The impasse frustrated Dan; shining a revealing light on the immortals was what he *did*. That Team Tiger wouldn't allow this added acid to the ink in a piece he wrote entitled "Nice (Not) Knowing You" for the February 2010 issue of *Golf Digest*, a couple of months after the fall. Here are two of the mildest paragraphs:

"I'll tell you what Hogan, Palmer and Nicklaus were at their peak," Jenkins wrote. "They were every bit as popular as Tiger, they endured similar demands on their time, but they handled it courteously, often with ease and enjoyment.

"They were never what Tiger allowed himself to be from the start: Spoiled, pampered, hidden, guarded, orchestrated, and entitled."

Four years later, Jenkins addressed his annoyance with his forced separation from about the only great golfer since Harry Vardon that he never interviewed by clacking out another write-around on his Olympia (a write-around, as you may recall, is a story or book executed without the co-operation of its subject; and an Olympia is a typewriter, an ancient mechanical device). This was the famous "My (Fake) Interview With Tiger":

Q. Why now?

A. Steinie says I have to rebuild my brand.

Q. Why? TV still loves you. The print press still loves you. The average fans still love you. Of course, the average fans still love the Kardashians, too, but I feel sure America will find a cure for this someday.

A. I just do what Steinie says.

Q. Why haven't you fired Steinie, by the way? You've fired everyone else. Three gurus, Butch, Hank, and Sean Foley. Two caddies, Fluff and Stevie. Your first agent, Hughes Norton, who made you rich before you'd won anything. Other minions.

A. I'll probably get around to it. I like to fire people. It gives me something to do when I'm not shaping my shots.

Q. Who would you rather run over in a car first, Brandel Chamblee or me?

A. Who's Brandel Chamblee? How many majors has he won? How many has he even *played*?

More years passed. Tiger got badly hurt and the world beat him down, but he came back; he continued to focus like a laser on winning; and he never lost his willingness to put in the practice tee reps to make it happen. Damn! Tiger had become more and more like Dan's dogged hero, Hogan. Post spinal-fusion surgery, he required his own version of the Hawk's long pre-game warmup. Hogan had to sit in an Epsom-salted tub for an hour before he could even think about playing a tournament round and he also often soaked his hands in ice water. He also sometimes drank ginger ale for its perceived diuretic effect. Tiger's regimen may also include a warm bath and icy marinade for the fingers. I don't know. He's not talking to me, either.

"You know, Dan never really met Tiger beyond a hand-shake," says Tarde. "I think that he was a little scared that Tiger was better than Hogan. I think in his heart of hearts he knew Tiger was better."

• • •

Patrick Reed couldn't believe how good it felt to be the king. "It was *awesome*," said the 2018 Masters champ of his return to the scene of his ascension. "I hadn't been back all year until Sunday"—when, as mentioned, he gave the kids a thrill at the Drive, Pitch, Putt competition just by being there. "Everyone saying 'Hey, Champ!' and my caddie getting bib number one. And then hosting the dinner on Wednesday. Ray Floyd, Gary, Jack, Mr. Watson . . ."

Mr. Watson is Tom, not Bubba. Although Bubba was there, too.

Reed attended Augusta State University. which has been re-named Augusta University, for some reason, and is just down Berckmans Road and then left on Walton Way from the National. The talented, extremely hard-working and focused young man led the Jaguars to two NCAA titles but, incredibly, and unfortunately, he received scant support from his hometown fans while winning the Masters. *That* blows!

"The feeling around the eighteenth green when he won was subdued to the point of being awkward," reported *GOLF Magazine*'s Alan Shipnuck a year ago. Because in a Montague and Capulet melodrama revolving around Reed's wife resulted in estrangement from his parents, who live in

Augusta, popular opinion was on the side of mom and dad and not the in-laws. But I didn't want to talk about that in our brief chat and I sensed or imagined Reed was relieved to leave the topic alone.

Toughest shots on the back nine?

"Well, twelve, of course. The wedge on fifteen if you lay up. And the tee ball on eighteen. You're coming out of a *chute*. It's easier with a hurting wind because you can just aim at the bunker . . . I tried drawing the ball (his natural spin) off that tee until my last three or four rounds when I went with the helicopter."

The chopper is Reed's block-out swing, an amusing, club twirling contortion he uses to prevent a hook. It's like Tiger's slider, but funnier.

Thank you, Patrick, and good luck, I said. The poor guy's gotten hammered because of his occasionally off-putting intensity and the family thing and for daring to copy you-know-who's Sunday ensemble of red shirt and black pants. Don't know if it's an homage or an in-your-face; the latter, I hope.

On this gray Monday morning six days before he and Reed would face the world in their competing red and black outfits, Tiger looked splendid in dove gray Nike Men's Flat Front Flex Pants and a Nike TW Vapor Mock Polo in a thought-provoking inky blue. With him out early were Justin Thomas and Fred Couples, wearing who cares. Tiger's clothes mattered because of apparel scripting, which is Nike letting retailers all over the world know in advance what Woods would wear each day—at least for the tournament rounds—the better to have the stuff in stock. For internet shoppers, of course, a new look was just a click away. The tournament shirts would be navy, gray, lilac, and fire engine. Just $85 a piece.

And this was clever: inside Tiger's Air Zoom TW71 shoes, right where the heels rest, Nike had compelled its manufacturer to reproduce an image of two praying hands, one in a golf glove. It was a humorous shout out to Amen Corner, the difficult three-hole stretch that starts the homeward nine at Augusta National. As in: I pray I make three pars. Amen.

Hewing to enthusiastic requests from the largest, happiest gallery on the property, Tiger, Justin, and Fred hit up on the par three sixteenth, then walked to the front of the tee, dropped another ball, and pulled out their lowest lofted irons. On the count of three, the trio simultaneously skipped shots off the pond's surface and up toward and even on the green: yet another tradition, and a fan favorite.

And the fans—sorry, patrons—clapped and yelled and walked along and looked into the sky and said: do not rain. Because their tickets had not been cheap. Those with the foresight to order early in the year paid about $450 for Monday and $750 for Tuesday. Wednesday tickets commanded a premium because another patron preference, the Par 3 tournament, takes place in the p.m. $1,500 for Wednesday. Prices rose as the date approached.

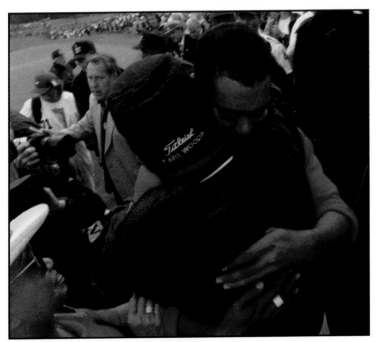

A family moment following the big win in the '97 Masters: Tida, Earl, Tiger.

(Dave Martin/Associated Press/AP Images)

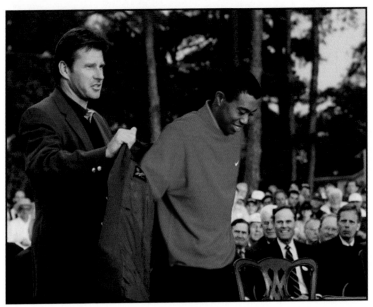

Welcome to the club. '96 champion Nick Faldo helps Woods
slip into a nice wool-polyester blend with two brass buttons.

(Amy Sancetta/Associated Press/AP Images)

Calvin Peete,
the best-ever
African-American
golfer until Tiger
came along, had an
inspirational backstory.

*(Lennox McLendon/Associated
Press/AP Images)*

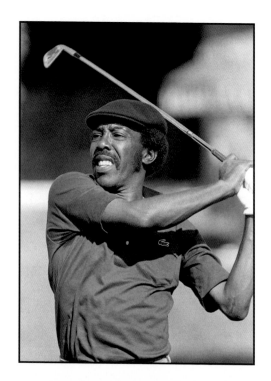

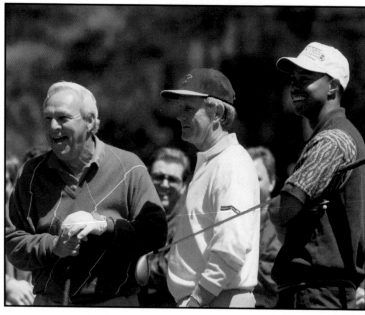

Among them, Arnie, Jack, and Tiger won the Masters fifteen times.

(Phil Sandlin/Associated Press/AP Images)

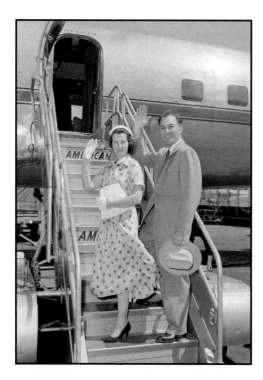

Valerie Hogan stood by her man at all times, including when he was in the hospital following their near-fatal car accident.

(Associated Press/AP Images)

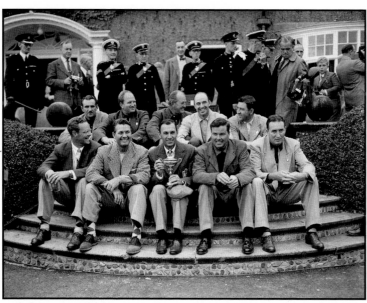

Skip Alexander—far left, front row—and the rest of the 1949 Ryder Cup team. Alexander survived a plane crash and burns over most of his body to make the team again in '51.

(Associated Press/AP Images)

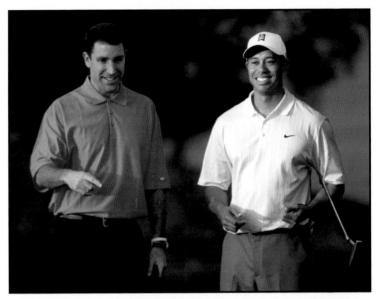

Agent Mark Steinberg made the deals and shooed away the press.

(Laurent Rebours/Associated Press/AP Images)

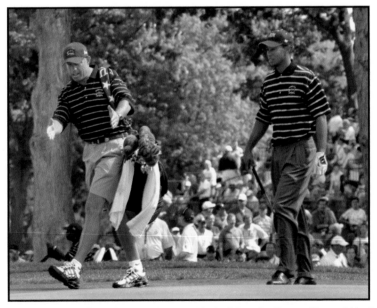

Caddie Steve Williams was an intense kind of Sancho Panza. He and Hank Haney left Team Tiger almost simultaneously in the wake of the sex scandal.

(James Marvin Phelps/Shutterstock.com)

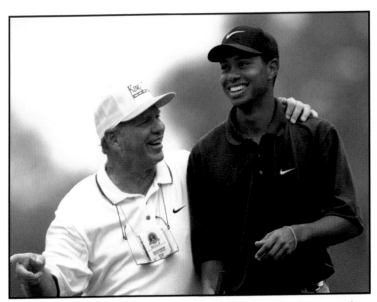

Instructor Butch Harmon would tell his successor "it's a tough team to be on."

(Dave Martin/Associated Press/AP Images)

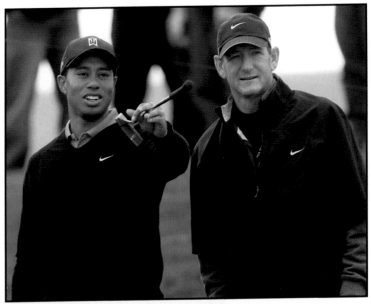

A tough team, indeed: Haney's book described the pleasure and pain of teaching the world's best golfer.

(Lenny Ignelzi/Associated Press/AP Images)

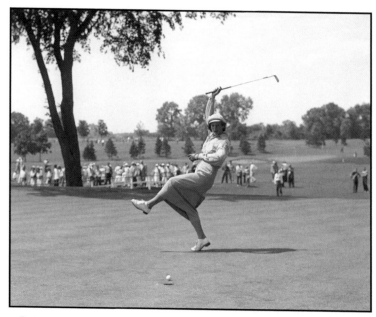

Between cancer surgeries, the charismatic Babe Didrikson Zaharias won the US Women's Open—by twelve shots.

(Ed Maloney/AP Images)

Six months after their wedding, Elin and Tiger embrace at the 2005 Masters. Their divorce became final in August 2010.

(Curtis Compton/Associated Press/AP Images)

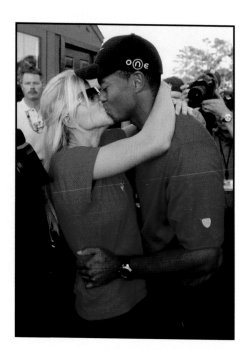

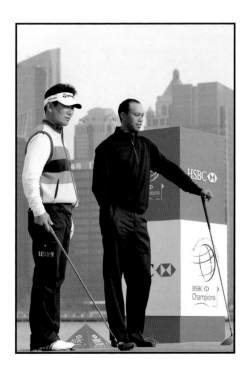

Y. E. Yang was on top of the world—and a skyscraper—following his shocking win over Tiger in the 2009 PGA Championship.

(Imaginechina-Editorial/Depositphotos.com)

The mighty Brooks Koepka spoke in epigrams and kept it simple. He fought Tiger to the wire in the '19 Masters.

(Chatchai Somwat/Shutterstock.com)

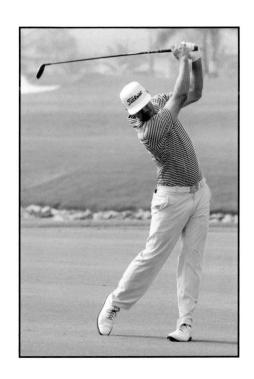

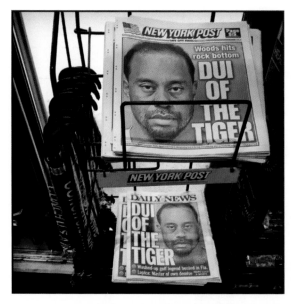

Page one of the New York City tabloids of May 29, 2017 differed only in their sub-heads: "Washed-up golf legend busted" for the *News* and "Woods hits rock bottom" for the *Post*.

(Courtesy of Mark Weinstein)

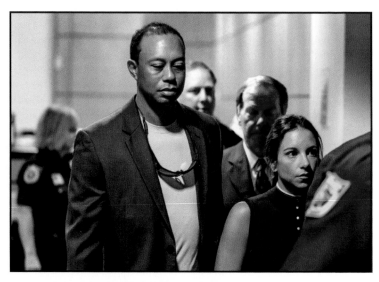

Tiger and girlfriend Erica Herman in a somber moment. But there were good times ahead.

(Lannis Waters/Associated Press/AP Images)

"Demand was about the same, maybe a little up from last year," says Clyde Pilcher, who virtually invented the Masters ticket re-selling business, and who remains one the biggest players in this game. "This year's Tuesday price was up a hundred dollars . . . Badges [good for Monday through Sunday] were $5,000 to $6,500.

"It's all corporate nowadays. Not many mom and pops buying badges because they're so expensive."

Pilcher, sixty-seven, was a poorer-than-poor Augusta kid whose all-encompassing work ethic made high school attendance an annoying hindrance to making money. At some point, Richmond Academy Assistant Principal Duford observed that because of all his absences, Clyde could get straight A's until kingdom come and still not graduate. OK, see ya, said the go-getter, well short of a diploma. He went to work, two jobs at a time. Among his employers were the City of Augusta Waterworks Department, Crane's Menswear, Borden's Ice Cream, three different gas stations, and Roto-Rooter. This last posting proved to be key because it inspired him to go out on his own. With a '61 Chevy C-10 pickup truck and a dream, Pilcher launched Budget Sewer Company. His big break was the big butter spill at the Murray Biscuit Company—which his competitors didn't want to mess with, and which Pilcher solved by cutting the handle off a shovel and going down deep in the clogged drain and digging it out himself. Soon Budget Sewer was living up to its slogan, "We're #1 in #2."

And this led to his Masters ticket business how?

"In '77 or '78 I was pumpin' out Mrs. Daisy Gallegos's septic tank at 301 Berckmans Road," a little house across the street from Gate 6 at Augusta National. "And she said she didn't want to fool with that house anymore. 'How much you want?' I asked. She says '$36,700.' I said, 'I'll take it.'"

Mrs. Clyde Pilcher questioned the wisdom of this purchase, but Clyde calculated that they'd make enough money parking cars to cover six of the $243.41 house payments to the mortgagor, the Bank of Texas.

"We got $2 a car, fifty cars at a time," Clyde recalls; when the competitor next door hired a cheerleader to attract customers, he got an even cuter cheerleader: his seven-year-old daughter, Traci. He just guided her curbside and put Richmond Academy purple pom-poms in her hands. *That's it honey, shake 'em!* And although the parking fees rose over the years from two to five to ten to twenty dollars per car, a new revenue stream soon dwarfed it.

Pilcher's lot was the perfect spot to connect patrons with what they wanted most. If a badge or a ticket needed to change hands, there was no need for the parties to work out the logistics for an in-person hand-off at Luigi's or at the Waffle House by the Bobby Jones Expressway; just put the coveted item in an envelope and leave it with Clyde. Both trading partners tipped the middleman, of course. Ten dollars here, twenty dollars there . . . One day Clyde rented an idle badge for a few hours to an antsy would-be patron for

$25. Eventually, he was buying and selling, but cautiously, only dealing with people he knew. And thus was born Badges Plus Inc.

"I'd been inside a septic tank for a twenty-five percent commission on a fifty-dollar sale," chuckles Pilcher. "But this shit was lucrative! I got so busy it was hard to park cars."

Clyde's eyes shine as he tells amazing stories from a life well lived; from glory days at Tubman Junior High to the Big Fight at Richmond Academy, a titanic, ten-minute tussle with Bill Paine—no relation to the Augusta National chairman of the same name—that ended in a tie; to all the adventure of being the more or less official Sewer Service of the Augusta National clubhouse and its cabins, and how all Budget Sewer services had to be performed at night because they couldn't take a chance on disturbing golfers with the sound of the pumps cleaning out the septic tanks; and how the end of the relationship illustrated the heavy-handed way the club sometimes dealt with its vendors. On a whim, it seemed, his invitation to play the Big Course on Vendor Day in May was withdrawn. Then find yourself another plumber, Clyde said.

"It cost them a fortune to replace us," he recalls. "Had to bring in someone from Atlanta. Next year, they dug up some fairways and tied into the city sewer line." There was the time a friend of his drove up with so much badge-related cash in his trunk—$150,000—that the poor man shook like a leaf on a tree and retired from the badge biz immediately and permanently. The canny Budget Sewer man developed a plan in case someone in his badge system died, and don't say it can't happen.

Almost without meaning to, Pilcher also became a flipper, buying and selling more parcels of real estate near the National, and he won big on that, too. "Paid $280,000 for those two lots," the poor boy who became a rich man says. "Sold them for three million . . ."

Back to badges: What does the ranking expert see for the market for the 2020 Masters?

"Next year? A lot depends on Tiger. If he's playin' good, I believe they will start at $8,000. Could be $10,000."

The face value of a badge in 2019, incidentally, was $375.

Shots having been skipped off pond water and their practice rounds complete, Woods, Couples, and Thomas retired from the scene. It began to rain. There was lightning. Patrons were ordered to leave.

Tuesday, April 9

The soothing pitter patter of rain on the roof did not tempt Tuesday's patrons to sleep in. Instead the $750 practice round watchers arrived like a waterproof army before sun-up in the cheerful April gloom, their car headlights bouncing off the black, rain-slick streets. They put on ponchos or opened umbrellas, made their way through the Masters' TSA-like check-in, then scarfed down a biscuit or bought some shirts and hats. There wasn't much golf to watch. At ten a.m., amidst a downpour and the threat of thunderstorms, play was suspended.

Woods would count it one of his best decisions all week that he did not play this day. Instead he stuck to the practice ground and did his drills and conserved energy. As he shared with Henni Zuel: "On Tuesday, when it just hosed down rain the course got opened up and all the guys who went out and played said it was useless to be out there because it was gonna be so much faster on Thursday."

With no practice round to play, father Tiger had a bit more time to play with his cubs. He was grateful, he said, to have Sam and Charlie with him, as they had been in Scotland the previous summer. "They were there when I failed," he said. "The last time they came out, I had a chance to win at the Open Championship. They felt the buzz of Dad on top of the board . . . and I lost. That sucked."

Failed, lost, sucked. This comment revealed something or reminded us of something important about Tiger. Perhaps the best way to understand him is as the special ops military man his father was and that he wanted to be. Missions were defined and they were completed, or they were not. When the mission is winning and you finish in a tie for sixth, then, well—you failed. Others could find something positive in a top ten in a major, but not this semi-SEAL.

With two holes remaining, Woods had been in with a chance against the infuriatingly steady Francesco Molinari, age thirty-five, a Euro Tour player who *never* seemed to make a bogey, and with whom Tiger was paired. Carnoustie looked like nuclear winter that week, as you may recall, what with its tan, drought-stricken fairways rolling as fast as Augusta National's sloping greens. Holes against the wind were tough as always, however, so Molinari, then tied for the lead with Xander Schauffele, had to stand on his two-iron second shot to the brutal seventeenth, the penultimate hole. And he nailed it. Tiger's second wasn't as good, nor was his attempt at a birdie, repeating the day's pattern. He trailed by two.

Eighteen—Jean van de Velde's Waterloo in the infamous Open of 1999—was just a drive and a flip on this day. With his rhythmic, tick-tock swing, Francesco hit a better drive than Tiger (although it must be said that some idiot yelled during the Woods backswing), a slightly better second, and he made his putt from six feet after Tiger missed his from seven. For the first time, an Italian man was the Champion Golfer of the Year.

Molinari!

Given that result and what was to occur two months later in France, Tiger could be forgiven for turning the name of his new nemesis into a curse. Just as Jerry Seinfeld's TV character disdained the one played by Wayne Knight—*Newman!*—the pleasant, well-liked *signore* from Turin must have crawled inside Tiger's skin.

After all the flag-raising and anthem playing and toasting to brotherhood and sportsmanship, the knives finally came out for the first matches in the Ryder Cup on September 28 at the Albatros course at Le Golf National in suburban Paris. In the first three matches, Team USA won, won, and won. The fourth match featured the American side's two fiercest competitors—Woods and Reed—versus the new Open champion and his partner, the long-haired Englishman, Tommy Fleetwood. Patrick and Tiger went two holes up, presaging a four to zero lead for the red, white, and blue, but Frankie and Tommy zoomed back to win the game 3 & 1. Team Europe won all four matches in the p.m.—a first in Ryder Cup history—with Molinari and Fleetwood spanking Justin Thomas and Jordan Spieth 5 & 4.

Captain Furyk put Reed/Woods out in the third match the next morning. And, *mon Dieu*, their opponents would be Molinari/Fleetwood again. There was the same infuriating result. Down eight points to four, Furyk chose a desperate course *après le déjeuner:* he would play his creaky, forty-two-year-old stud a second time, and let's just hope his vertebrae don't come unbolted. For a shot of youthful exuberance, Captain Jim paired Tiger with Ryder Cup rookie Bryson DeChambeau, age twenty-five.

If you don't already know, you can guess who the opponents were, and you can guess who won.

Molinari!

Fleetwood got thrashed by Tony Finau in the singles on Sunday but his fourball and foursomes partner won again, becoming the first-ever European player to score the maximum five points. Counting the Open, Francesco had Molinaried Tiger's ass four times in two months.

He was a hard man to dislike, however, no matter what flag you stood under. He had a sense of humor: Francesco and Tommy produced a fifty-two-second video that showed them lying in bed with the Ryder Cup between them the morning after . . . whatever. How was it for you? Francesco asks. Tommy replies, "I'd give you five out of five, Frankie."

Every member of both Ryder Cup teams toiled during the Tuesday practice session. Woodstock-level mud marred the high traffic areas on the course. Squeegee teams worked overtime. Practice tee instructors studied their clients' swings as if they were defusing bombs. But some of the gentlemen had to cut their exertions short. Woods, Reed, Spieth, Phil Mickelson, Bubba Watson, and Sergio Garcia all had to get ready for dinner.

They returned to the club freshly showered and almost identically dressed, all the former champions having faced the annual question: what color tie best complements a green jacket? Mickelson ('06, '10) selects red for tonight; Nicklaus ('63, '65, '66, '72, '75, '86) always chooses yellow. There's that adverb again.

The Champions Dinner is a time capsule or a funeral rehearsal, but with cocktails and more laughs. Craig Stadler ('82) now looks like Wilford Brimley. José-María Olazábal ('94, '99) emanates a Most Interesting Man in the World vibe. Without a Nike Aerobill Classic 99 hat on his head,

Tiger Woods ('97, '01, '02, '05) reminds that male pattern baldness runs in families, and that time flies.

The Dinner was started by Ben Hogan in '52, in gratitude for his win in '51, after near misses in '42—a playoff loss to Byron Nelson—and '46—a three-putt on the final green that put Herm Keiser's long arms into a green jacket. At first it was just the defending champ picking up the tab for the former champs but at some point, the defender began to pick the bill of fare, too—although going off-menu has never been a problem. Sandy Lyle ('88), a Scot, presented haggis as a starter in '89. "I didn't eat that," recalled Charles Coody ('71). "I knew what it was."

The club gives the participants two clubhouse badges and pays them an honorarium large enough for Coody to at least feign an interest in boiled sheep guts mixed with onions and oatmeal.

Curiosity about the menu is always high. Tiger showed that he was still just a kid when he featured cheeseburgers and milkshakes in 1998. Reed mandated more nuanced flavors in '19. "I'm definitely going to fatten everyone up," he announced, and then he showed how. The entrée would be bone-in ribeye with herb butter. Sides were mac and cheese, creamed spinach, and corn crème brûlée. The wines were Napa Valley Chardonnay and Cab. Among the dessert options were chocolate crunch and praline cheesecake.

1971 champ Charles Coody chose the healthy entrée

option, mountain trout, and it was good. The whole evening was good. But it was not an especially fun or entertaining interval because the current roster lacks a storyteller to spin a post-prandial tale or two. Claude Harmon, Jimmy Demaret, Gene Sarazen, Henry Picard, and especially Sam Snead could be counted on for funny or revealing anecdotes and dirty jokes—read: Snead—but they are all gone now. Jack Burke, Jr. loves to declaim and he can be a spellbinder, but he is ninety-six now and hasn't been back to Augusta for several years.

What about Tiger?

"Tiger doesn't talk much," said Coody. "But it seems like he's flipped over a new leaf. He's a little bit more approachable. I think he's matured quite a bit."

The Dinner got tiresome, eventually, for some of the oldsters. Maybe everything does. "It used to be fun," Sarazen ('34) told me in '97, when he was ninety-five. "But now the room's too small. There's too many of them (other former Masters champs) and they all want hats and everything else signed so they can take them back to their clubs and sell 'em."

As Burke told Murray of *The Guardian* a few years ago, "What happens is you get to where you don't even know the players. I won't go back. It's too hard. You have to drive 150 miles (from Atlanta) for one dinner. I don't see the reason for it now."

And yet it is the one meal every player yearns to eat.

Wednesday, April 10

Gilbert A. Freeman, the Director of Golf at Lakewood Country Club in Dallas, yields to no man in his love for the Masters. He'd as soon give up brisket enchiladas as miss April in Augusta and *that* ain't gonna happen. He feels similarly about Eldrick T. Woods: loves his flair, his look, his demeanor, and his achievement. And Gilbert puts his money where his mouth is, by stocking the Lakewood golf shop with plenty of Nike.

"I sat behind him on the range on Wednesday and watched him hit balls, like I always do," Freeman recalls. "He was ripping it. A laser light show. Never missed a shot. Later, I was on the phone to my members. 'Bet on Tiger,' I said.

"He seems to be instructor-free now. This new guy, Matt Killen, really looks to be just be an extra set of eyes."

Tiger stopped hitting, made eye contact with his mates, and the four of them walked from the range behind the clubhouse to the tenth tee. "I followed him out onto the course for his nine-hole practice round with Couples, Kevin Kisner, and Justin Thomas," Freeman testifies. "And he was smiling and jacking around and still just *killing* the ball. He was way less tense than I'd ever seen him."

These four had to finish by one o'clock, because the Big Course, as members call it, would close, as always, for final primping, while the attention turned to the little course. No one calls it that; it's the Par 3 Golf Course and it is the living legacy of club and tournament co-founder Cliff Roberts, even though Cliff shot and killed himself by the banks of one of its two ponds on a black night seventeen years after it opened for business.

From the Masters debut in 1934 until 1959, the club had presented various activities on the day or days leading up to the tournament. Long driving contests were a staple; a big old boy named George Bayer usually won. At least once they had a bow and arrow exhibition. The first Masters Festival parade in 1957 rolled down Broad Street downtown and had about what you'd expect: marching bands, floats, and golf pros waving to the fans—are they still patrons when they're off campus?—25,000 of them that first year, according to the *Chronicle*, with the golf heroes riding in white Oldsmobile and Cadillac convertibles. Miss Golf Pageant contestants competed in gown, swimsuit, talent, and three-putt avoidance. We're kidding about the three-putt thing, but the club had a deep desire to attract and keep fans back in the day when the golf alone was not enough to ensure the tournament's survival.

Augusta National's benign dictator decided to try something else as well. In a letter to the membership in 1958, Roberts proposed building a par 3 course with an estimated cost of $67,500. Subscription forms enclosed. Although he was no architect, Roberts rode herd on the thing so hard he deserves a co-designer credit with George Cobb. It was an incredible success. From its opening in 1960, the Par 3 was a hit, providing a fun, fast way for members and their guests to warm up for or cool down from a round on the Big Course. And on Wednesday of Masters Week, the Par 3 would provide light-hearted competition for former champs and current competitors on holes that currently range from seventy-seven yards up to 151. With images of pink and white flowering dogwoods and colorfully dressed patrons bouncing off the surface of its two reflecting ponds, the Par 3 is a little sliver of golf heaven. There's no room, so spectators don't move around; they just find a spot and sit there.

"It used to be fun, and then they stopped selling beer," muses local raconteur Tim Wright. "Now you have to walk all the way over to the concession area by the main entrance, get you two beers, and they're gone by the time you're back to the Par 3. They want a family atmosphere, I guess. They can have it."

Family it is. Wives, girlfriends, kids, and Patton Kizzire's mama looked impossibly cute in their white caddie jumpsuits and green caps. Matt Wallace, an English pro from suburban London, won in a playoff with Sandy Lyle—a footnote. Oddly, for the second consecutive year, a tall Polynesian Mormon grabbed the Par 3 spotlight from the adorable kids and the gracious legends.

As you may recall from April of '18: Masters rookie Milton Pouha "Tony" Finau strode to the eighth tee with, we think, the largest entourage of any player. Arrayed around him as he selected a gap wedge for the 121-yard shot were his lovely wife Alayna and the couple's four young children.

Team Finau jumped and shouted along with everyone else when dad spun his shot into the hole. Tony, too. He flung his club in the air, ran forward twenty or thirty yards in exaltation—a good high school hoopster, he is quite light on his feet—pirouetted to look at Alayna and the kids and then, in the midst of this crazy celebration: down goes Finau!

The video went bacterial. Past viral.

Almost as quickly as Finau dislocated his ankle, he relocated it. Alayna rushed to her stricken husband. "Oh my gosh, dude," she said. "Did you really just pop your ankle back in place?" He had and it hurt like hell but he wobbled through the final Par 3 hole then asked his agent to find him an orthopedist, a magnetic resonance imaging machine, and an aspirin. It would be a shame for anyone to miss the Masters in such a bizarre (yet amusing) mishap, of course. But if Finau did have to send his regrets in the morning, his thoughts would surely turn to Tiger and to April 1997.

Tony, then age seven, sat on the couch in the Finaus' crowded house that cold weekend in Salt Lake City, transfixed by the TV. He'd never watched a golf tournament before this moment. "I saw this kid who was the same color as me," he would recall. "At the exact moment I started out, I watched Tiger Woods win the Masters. The way he fist-pumped, the red shirt, his power compared to the other players, the way he made the fans go crazy, and the rawness of it all seemed larger than life.

"I looked at it and I'm like, man, maybe I can do that someday, maybe I can play in the Masters . . . [but] I didn't dream of just playing in the Masters, I dreamed of winning it."

"It's impossible to overestimate Tiger's influence on kids like me, or the impact he's had on golf in general."

Kelepi, Tony's father, was from the Kingdom of Tonga, a remote Pacific island nation that is a world leader in corruption and obesity. He moved to the US with his family at age eleven. He met and married Ravena, also Polynesian, and somehow kept his family afloat on the $35,000 Delta and Western Airlines paid him for handling its baggage. And while Kelepi Finau didn't know from golf, he was an excellent athlete who understood how sports can keep kids too busy for trouble. And there was trouble outside the doors in their poor neighborhood in the form of easy access to drugs and gangs. A lot of Pacific Islanders had coalesced in Salt Lake City; so had the Tongan Crip Gang, the Sons of Samoa, and other similar youth groups up from LA. The Finau boys would not be joining.

Kelepi sought out Salvation Army clubs and scrounged for golf balls. He checked out *Golf My Way* from the library and painstakingly absorbed Jack Nicklaus's instructional wisdom. And he placed strips of carpet on the floor of the garage and hung an old mattress from the ceiling joists. Tony hit from the rug on one side, and his younger brother from the other, aiming at spray painted targets that were low, medium, and high. When the Utah weather warmed up, the

Finau brothers, Gipper and Tony, wore out the practice green at a nearby par three course. They didn't play because they couldn't afford a green fee.

"We hit thousands and thousands of chips, maybe millions," Tony said. "We learned what it was like to make the right sound when you make a solid chip at Jordan River par 3 course."

A turning point arrived, and not an unusual one in golf, thank goodness: the pro, Richard Mason, recognizing their talent and drive, started to let the brothers play for free. Out on the course, Tony discovered the ferocity of Jordan River mosquitos, which led him to wear high socks and to play fast, habits he took into adulthood. Now, many years later, he stood on one foot on the brink of his childhood goal, with the other foot swelling and turning purple.

He played anyway—with a limp—and cemented his legend, shooting 68-74-73-66, tied for tenth, far behind the standard set by the winner, Reed, but good enough for an invitation to return.

Given his wipeout the previous year, no one would have blamed Finau if he gave the Par 3 a pass in 2019. Instead, he and his agency, Wasserman, and his equipment company, Nike, produced a mockumentary on the development of the Nike Finau1, footwear to prevent celebration-related ankle injuries. They released the video just before the Masters. It's pretty good; there's plenty of deadpan dialogue from the star. "I'm most proud of having a shoe that can help others," Tony says. "And when they make a hole-in-one, and it's time to celebrate, they know which shoe to wear."

Everyone got the joke. The big ugly green Finau1 golf boot on Tony's left foot got a laugh on every hole.

Thursday, April 11

9:58   Finau, Sergio Garcia, Henrik Stenson

11:04   Woods, Jon Rahm, Haotong Li

1:16   Molinari, Rafa Cabrera-Bello, Tyrrell Hatton

2:00   Koepka, Jordan Spieth, Paul Casey

In the dawn's early light, hours before Tony, Tiger, Frankie, and Brooks sucked in cleansing breaths and took aim at the green, green grass to the left of the blindingly white granulated quartz fairway bunker, out strode the Honorary Starters.

After a fulsome introduction, TV news anchor-haired Augusta National Chairman Fred Ridley said, "Ladies and gentlemen, from South Africa, Gary Player." The little man in black, age eighty-three, looked terrific. He has been a fitness fiend and out there about it his whole life. "Feel that stomach!" he has said to many an amazed stranger. "Like iron!" And sometimes people obliged him with the poke he wanted—but uneasily, I think, from the times I've seen it done.

Player swatted a ball up the fairway with a reasonable facsimile of the swing that won the Masters three times.

The years have been less kind to the GOAT. Jack Nicklaus, seventy-nine, the greatest of all-time in terms of majors won—eighteen—and Masters won—six, is drooping and stooping, the effect of extra weight and osteoarthritis. The Golden Bear in a yellow sweater slapped one up the middle well short of Gary's ball, waved his hand dismissively at his effort, and the 2019 Masters had launched.

Which was just the word for what was to occur on the tee of the first hole and every other par four and par five, because to observe, for example, Finau and Koepka hitting a driver was to witness a suborbital trip toward the stratosphere. That the ball goes a good deal farther than it used to is not in dispute but what to do about it is. As the owners of one fourth of golf's majors and about half its traditions, the members of Augusta National have been particularly irked and discommoded by golf's inability to control its distance fetish. All other games have an official ball but it's good for business for golf ball manufacturers to have sliced and diced the pill into various permutations of spin and flight, and of compounds, construction, and color, and now we're sure we need them all.

How about a special dead Masters ball? That might connect the tournament to its past. But Chairman Ridley, the 1975 US Amateur champ, who was also USGA president, shot down the idea in his annual (since 2017) address to the press. The club will, apparently, keep adding length and planting trees. For example: the forty yards added to the fifth for 2019 made an already tough hole brutal. Now the landing area for drives on this 495-yard par four is a resistant upslope and the green is crazy.

With its recent purchase of acreage from its Rae's Creek neighbor, Augusta Country Club, Augusta National might even add length to its thirteenth, one of the best and most famous holes in the game, but the easiest hole in the Masters.

"Is your course long enough yet?" I asked an insider.

"I don't know," he, or possibly she, said. "Right now we're waiting to see if the USGA or the R&A or the PGA Tour are gonna do anything about the ball."

A few years ago, Lee Trevino dumbed it all down for me: trampoline effect, spin rates, the cubic centimeters in driver heads, and golf giving the finger to the curve-it-left, bend-it-right shot maker game he played. Blame the USGA, not Augusta National, Trevino said.

"They complain that the Masters is making the course too long. But do you think people want to see Tiger Woods hit a three-iron off every tee? That patron ain't gonna pay [a small fortune] to see that. He wants the homerun ball.

"What they should do is increase the diameter of the ball to 1.72 and take an eighth of an ounce off."

Had Nicklaus and Woods sat together at the Dinner the night before, they might have had that conversation. Jack's been vocal about reeling in the ball for many years. When Tiger won the Open at the Old Course at St. Andrews in 2005, he flew his tee balls over bunkers that had been ensnaring golfers for centuries. More proof that something ain't right, Jack said; when he'd won the Open at St. Andrews in 1970 and 1978, he was by far the strongest man in golf, but those sand pits had been in play for him.

After a life of silence on the subject, Tiger caused a kerfuffle in November '17 when he said: "We need to do something about the golf ball. I just think it's going too far . . . I think the 8,000-yard golf course is not too far away. And that's pretty scary because we don't have enough property to start designing these type of golf courses and it just makes it so much more complicated."

Up stepped an argument for the five-mile golf course.

"Ladies and gentlemen, the 9:58 starting time," called out the starter. "Fore, please. Tony. Finau. Now drivin'."

After his early years banging balls into a bed and playing the game on a teeny-weenie par 3, pre-teen Tony finally got to stretch out in the wider open spaces of regulation-length golf courses. He shocked people with how far he hit it. At age ten, he could blast a driver 240 yards.

How he did it also amazed. Picture, for a moment, notoriously long hitters like John Daly and virtually everyone in a long drive competition: at the top of their backswings their hands are behind their necks. Their swings describe a circle and a half. But Finau saves himself time and complication by barely getting his hands above his pants pockets going back before crashing into the ball. Was there a low ceiling in that garage? His swing looks entirely composed of follow-through. Yet some weeks he's the biggest hitter in the tournament; in this Masters, he'd average about 320. When

Tony catches one with his Ping the ball seems to hang in the air as if it were weightless, or a drone flying away.

"Fore, please. Tiger. Woods. Now drivin'.'"

Jon Rahm, Haotong Li, and Tiger have already observed the scorecard trading and golf ball identifying ritual. "TaylorMade . . . Pro V . . . Bridgestone," they murmur. Rahm and Woods will both play the TaylorMade M5 driver with Speed Injected Twist Face Technology. Li will go into battle with the M6 with Speed Injected Twist Face Technology, putting him one M up.

Tiger stands behind the ball, picturing the perfect shot, his mind closed to the stimuli from the huge adhesive crowd. At some point today—when he got up? On the range? Just now?—gallons of concentration and focus have poured over him, like syrup on a waffle. His face has become a mask. To me, at least, the mask resembles the face of Toshiro Mifune, the handsome Japanese actor who could *do* intense.

Woods wears, as promised, the navy shirt. "Think about those clothes for a second," offers Tommy Brannen, the pro at Augusta Country Club. "When Tiger started, golf shirts were huge. Now, because of him, they're much tighter. They show off your muscles—if you have them."

Tiger has them. His mind made up, he steps forward— right foot, left foot, right, left. He takes one last look and then he swings.

"Fore, please. Francesco. Molinari. Now drivin'.'"

A normally shaped man of 1.7 meters and 72 kilograms,

Open champion Molinari recalls the day when the best golfers in the world were five-eight, one-sixty (or passing through one-sixty) and they didn't lift weights. The best examples are the game's Mount Rushmore figures—Hogan, Nicklaus, Palmer, and Jones—who were good but not great athletes who mastered the ball and mastered themselves. The awesome physiques of Dustin Johnson, Koepka, Tiger, Henrik Stenson, and other current players make us overestimate the importance of height, clubhead speed, and time in the forty. Especially at the elite level, the strongest mind wins.

The stories on most pens and in most media mouths this Masters Week had been the possibilities of Tiger, of course, and the body of Brooks Koepka, because there was a lot less of it and people wanted to know why on earth there was less. He'd lost about twenty-five pounds, Brooks said, but he didn't share his motivation. When he got some stick for it in his presser after the first round, he responded with haiku-like simplicity:

"I lift too many weights and I'm too big to play golf.

"And then when I lose weight, I'm too small.

"I'm going to make me happy. I don't care what anyone else says.

"I'm doing it for me, and obviously it seems to work."

Obviously: he'd just shot sixty-six and was tied for the lead after the first round of the Masters. After a front nine that was mere preamble, the nerveless, gifted athlete birdied five out of six, starting with the dead-easy twelfth; just a three-quarter nine iron and a putt from the fringe. It was a good time to be Brooks. The geometrical, symmetrical former Florida State Seminole had surged to number one in the world and was still rising, because in the previous three US Opens, he'd finished first, first, and second, and in the last two PGA Championships, first and first. What an unbelievable resume he suddenly had, what a life he was living. If we were having cocktails, I'd ask him about being the 2004 Sir Henry Cotton Rookie of the year on the European Tour. And possibly about his fit and photogenic girlfriend, Ms. Jena Sims, who had had a featured role in *Sharknado 5: Global Swarming.*

Tiger shot seventy, two under, and liked it. "I've shot this number and won four coats so hopefully I can do it again," he said. In truth, only three of his four wins had started with seven oh. He'd dialed the wrong number with a first round seventy-four in 2005 but then set the world right by finishing with sixty-six, sixty-five, seventy-one, enough to force a playoff with Chris DiMarco, you may recall, which Tiger won. That had been his last win in Augusta—fourteen years ago, but it seemed even farther in the past than that.

Steady Molinari birdied fifteen and eighteen to tie Woods with seventy.

Finau shot seventy-one. He didn't wear the boot.

Night fell and wonderful times were had all over town. Clouds and cooler air blew in gently from the north and the west.

Friday, April 12

10:09	Molinari	70	
11:04	Koepka	66	T-1
12:54	Finau	71	
1:49	Woods	70	

Don M. Wilson III put his 2004 BMW 330ci in gear and Greenwich in his rearview mirror. With his hands at ten and two and the radio tuned to Motown and BBC podcasts of "In Our Time," he rolled south at all deliberate speed from Connecticut through New York City, Jersey, and Philly on I-95, the longest north-south road in the USA and the fourth-busiest interstate in the country. The MapQuest directions couldn't have been simpler: get on I-95 and go south for 777 miles. Exit at Bull Street. And, bam, you're there, "there" for the tired retired banker being the Comfort Inn in Columbia, South Carolina. Winter still gripped the country that Wilson left early that Tuesday morning but in the capital of the Palmetto State warm air and dots and blots of pink, red, and white bloomers signaled spring. The drive had taken eleven hours and change.

Wilson rendezvoused with his son, Rob, an Indiana U. grad now getting another degree at the Johns Hopkins University School of Advanced International Studies, who flew in from D.C. early the next morning. The airport in Columbia is on the west side of town; it's only a one-hour drive to Augusta. The Wilsons had tickets to the Par 3.

"Wonderful," Wilson said afterward. "A terrific concept. You're really close to the players. Very relaxed, not a competitive feel to it."

That Wilson had never been to the Masters before seemed odd, for seldom will you find a more enthusiastic and hooked-up golfer, or one less tolerant of dithering during a round. DMW3, as his friends call him, plays to an eight at a race walk. An Anglophile, he's attended "at least twenty" Open Championships. In addition to membership at such gemlike courses as The Sand Hills in Nebraska and Garden City in New York, Wilson expresses his love for the game by publishing weird, wonderful books about it. The ninth and latest slip-cased, limited edition offering from Grant Books—H.R.J. Grant of Droitwich, Worcestershire, England, is Wilson's publishing partner—is called *Machrihanish: Machaire Shanais Golf 1880s-1920s*. Machrihanish is an achingly lovely links course in a remote corner of Scotland; *machaire shanais* is Scottish Gaelic for "plain of whispers." My copy of Grant & Wilson's *Edwardian Golf Library 1900-1914* stays open to Chapter Six, "Poetry and Songs."

Like every other Augusta National virgin, the Wilsons were awed by what they saw on Thursday and Friday.

"It's one of the greatest outdoor spaces in the world," said DMW3. "It's a horticultural gem that happens to have a golf course that happens to be really good . . . Not many spectator stands compared to an Open and far fewer people. I loved the no-cell-phones policy and the non-digitized scoreboards and their relative scarcity. They have live radio at an Open but not at Augusta. But it's fun to not know the score sometimes . . . It's over-staffed, which is wonderful. The workers make you feel like you're their guest, a guest of a family and not of a corporation."

Koepka birdied the first hole, then hit a big old hook off two, into a heavily treed area that golfer/comedians from an earlier era called "the Delta ticket counter"—the obvious joke being that finding oneself left on two leads to an early flight out of Augusta, Columbia, or Atlanta. Brooks double bogeyed the seventh hole and was two over for the day after six but rallied a bit and finished with a seventy-one and a tie for the lead.

Afterward, there was more haiku from Koepka:

"There's no point in getting too excited on a Friday.

"You've still got a lot of golf to play, so you've just got to hang in there."

Molinari led with a few others. His sixty-seven—composed of thirteen pars and five birdies—included a deuce on the easy twelfth. The steady excellence of his play at the Open, in the most recent Ryder Cup, and this week in Augusta, was giving him an aura of unflappability that turned the national stereotype on its ear. He was not the tenor in the opera but the ticket taker out front. Not a hot-blooded and mercurial Latin man but an unassuming and self-contained strategist—a Russian chess champion, maybe?

Molinari didn't have the personality for it, really, but he and Tiger had at least a little bit of a rivalry as we mentioned. They'd met cute, as they say in Hollywood. Francesco and his brother Edoardo had made a pact that whichever of the two qualified for the Masters first would have the other brother for a caddie. Edoardo won the 2005 US Amateur, which got him an invitation to Augusta, a pairing for the first two rounds with the defending champion—Tiger—and a sherpa he'd known all his life.

"After a few holes both Tiger and Steve Williams went to my brother and asked him, 'There's a guy playing on the European tour [who's] playing well with a name similar to yours' and my brother is like, 'Yeah, he's my brother.'

"'Is he playing this week? What's he doing?'

"My brother says, 'No, no he's over there. With the white overalls.'"

It was not a great experience for Francesco. "I didn't really enjoy caddying," he recalled. "It seemed a bit of a nightmare, standing with the bag, waiting for him to hit the shots. It's not great fun to caddie around here."

Unspoken by the polite Molinari were two other things that make carrying a bag in the Masters a beat-down: the hills, and those damn oven-like coveralls. It's past time for a miracle fabric, or a completely new look—perhaps culottes.

Molinari's game progressed nicely if not dramatically. In 2010, he warranted his first invitations to the Masters— he finished 30th—and to Europe's Ryder Cup team. He played against Tiger in the Sunday singles. The American won but America lost. At the next Cup, the 2012 edition at Medinah Country Club in suburban Chicago, Francesco's *sang froid*—*in italiano, a sangue freddo*—earned him the most nervous-making slot in the batting order, the final match on the final day. He'd play against Tiger yet again.

In what was either the most epic meltdown in Ryder Cup history or its most stirring comeback, Team Europe climbed back from a four-point deficit to win the Match. Woods and Molinari tied theirs. No one spoke of a blooming rivalry.

Back at the Masters, and as for Finau: no one but friends and family noticed him shoot seventy-one on Friday. But: patience. On Saturday he would set this world on fire.

Tiger teed off at 2:18, a half hour later than scheduled. The field's pokiness was due to drizzly weather. He'd been up for a while; his day had started when it was still dark as night. While the others in his luxurious rental house at The River Golf Club lay in bed, presumably, Tiger had lifted his Titleist Scotty Cameron Newport 2 putter from his Monster Energy golf bag—he never stores his clubs at the course—signaled "walk time" to the dog, and man and beast slipped out the door.

The pawprints and footprints in the dew showed that they walked across a fairway bordering the road and then to a green, where Tiger did what he does: he rolled some putts. A couple of maintenance workers drove up to investigate the shadowy golfer in the starless night. "He couldn't have been nicer," says Chris Verdery, the club's Director of

Golf. "They just talked about his late starting time that day and they took a few selfies. I like that he just acted like a regular guy. He obviously wasn't really practicing, because we've got Bermuda greens and Augusta National has bentgrass."

And yet: Tiger would roll in, let's see . . . 132 feet of birdie putts this day, including increments of twenty-five, thirty, and thirty-seven. The made long putt had been a staple of his game back in his heyday; had those glorious old days returned? He was getting standing ovations on almost every green, just for being Tiger. When he finished his round with a sixty-eight that put him within a shot of the lead, it was the closest he'd been to the halfway lead at the Masters in fourteen years. Enthusiasm for the magnetic man only increased now that he was in it with a chance to win it.

He was the People's Champ. Despite Molinari, DJ, Koepka, Rose, Rory, and Spieth; despite the back, the past, and the passage of time; despite everything, and until further notice, Tiger was the king.

How did he look? we asked a witness.

"Utterly composed," replied DMW3.

Saturday, April 13

1:15 p.m.	Finau	70-71=141	
2:05	Woods	70-68=138	T-6
2:30	Koepka	66-71=137	T-1
2:45	Molinari	70-67=137	T-1

• • •

Donna Archer arrived early, as she always had, and walked Augusta National backwards, from eighteen to one, also same as always. Along the way during the week she'd said hi to the usual people, dear old friends she saw only once a year lately: Tom Watson, Gary Player, the Langers, the Coodys, the Norths, the Azingers, Jack and Barb Nicklaus. Mrs. Archer is a lively, upbeat woman but this year she felt the sweet weight of nostalgia more than usual, for this tournament marked the fiftieth anniversary of her late husband's unlikely win in the 1969 Masters, over several better-known competitors, especially Tom Weiskopf and Billy Casper. Tom, by the way, would be a four-time Masters runner-up; Billy won the tournament the next year.

Mrs. Archer came to the twelfth hole and paused for a moment.

"George always played twelve very conservatively. It wasn't a notable hole for him," Donna recalled. "But he was paired with Weiskopf—or was in the group right behind him—when Tom put a hundred balls in the water."

It wasn't a hundred. But full-immersion baptism of five balls in Rae's Creek and a couple of putts added up to a double-quintuple, I guess you'd call it—a ten-over 13. Amen, Corner, and let us pray. We've said jokingly that twelve is easy but, as everyone knows, it's not easy, partly because the air above it swirls like a banana in a blender. And the wind isn't the only thing that makes this 155-yard pitch to a patch of green ice one of the hardest holes on the course. It's proven far harder to par than the famed island green seventeenth at TPC Sawgrass.

The stories you hear . . . imagine that the next two victims tell their tales while shining a flashlight under their respective chins on a dark, dark night:

"It was a Friday, and I was playing pretty well, and I looked OK with the cut," said D.A. Weibring. "Then, I got to twelve. The wind was against, the pin was back. I hit a six iron which hit six feet from the pin, released, and rolled into the back bunker. Now I've got the hardest shot in the world, downhill lie, downhill shot, no green, and Rae's Creek waiting for me. Long story short, I made a six-footer for an eight."

The night is silent but for the crackle and pop from the campfire. Overcome, Weibring hands the torch to Bob Gilder.

"The first year my son ever caddied for me, I was one shot off the lead on the second day." The light briefly sparkles off the shine in Gilder's eyes. "On the back nine, I kept hitting good shots that just didn't work out. A bogey on eleven, then a seven or an eight on the par three . . ."

Just as rain falls equally on the just and the unjust, even the greatest among us have had to put up with mockery from the twelfth hole. With five shots in hand and just nine to play in 2016, Jordan Spieth bogied ten and eleven—not fatal, and not unusual—but he hit his nine iron at the back right flag on twelve and didn't make it. Then he dropped a ball, tried again, and didn't make it. The resultant quadruple bogey seven enabled an unlikely win for Danny Noonan—no, sorry, Danny *Willett*. His only on the PGA Tour as of this writing.

One year in the '60s, the crusty old green-jacketed co-founders rolled down the hill in a cart to watch Jones favorite Jack Nicklaus play number twelve, which was a big deal because Bobby was mortally ill with a neurological disease and was getting out of his cabin less and less every year. Jack saw Jones and Roberts parked off to the side. The very large crowd grew silent. Jack went through the stations of his intricate pre-shot routine. At last the deliberate golfer swung—and whistled a shank right over Cliff's and Bobby's heads.

Donna Archer completed her backward tour of the cathedral in the pines and thought of her late husband. On another sunny day fifty Aprils before, George Archer, the tallest-ever major winner and one of the game's best putters, shrugged his way into a 42L and the people cheered.

On her long walk she'd passed our *dramatis personae* while they were shooting sixty-four (Finau), sixty-six (Molinari), a sixty-seven for Tiger, and sixty-nine for Koepka. Fantastic stuff! And time for some italics.

Finau *nearly eagled three holes* on the front nine, having lipped out a bunker shot on two, a pitch on three, and then, on eight, the uphill, left-bending, hardest par five on the course—Tony made history. Almost. On this same hole fifty-two Masters before, Bruce Devlin espied a good lie for his Dot just in the right rough. The Aussie had 248 yards to the unseen flagstick. He took a lusty cut with a wooden four wood, hit a hook, and damned if the ball didn't roll in.

That was 1967. In 2019, on what is now a much longer hole, Finau had 230 yards to the front edge, and 261 to the pole—"a comfortable four iron for me," he said. He pured it, as they say, and his ball almost did a Devlin, stopping a baby's foot away. After the tap-in eagle, he had a ten-footer on nine for a twenty-nine, which would have been the lowest-ever first half score in Masters history—but this time his Bettinardi Precision Milled Putter was a fraction off.

When he met the press a few hours later, the talk was of the unprecedentedly early start planned for Sunday, due to looming bad weather late in the afternoon, and of the possibility of his being paired with Tiger.

"It would be an unbelievable thing for me . . . a dream come true for me," Tony said, but he didn't seem as awed as his words implied. Because, on the other hand: "Tiger taught us how to compete. You shouldn't fear anybody. He's playing against guys he kinda bred."

For about eighteen minutes, Finau really leaned into the questions asked, a compliment to the askers; his effort to understand, his disarming style, and a frequent smile made him easily the best of The Four at the media give-and-take.

"Being Tongan and Samoan is a huge part of who I am,"

he said in response to a question seldom asked in polite company. "We're driven people. We're also very relaxed. I like to have a good time on the golf course."

When Molinari salvaged a par on the eighteenth with a sublime long bunker shot, it was his *forty-third hole in a row without a bogey.* The "clean card" was important to him; during his brief interrogation he evinced more pride in his par putts on four and five than on the six birdies he'd made.

You have a two-shot lead, Francesco. What will be your plan for tomorrow?

Plan! Molinari smirked at the very idea. "There gonna be a few guys trying to mess up with my plan," he said. He's monotone in his second language, and he seemed weary, as well—after all the hillwalking, concentration, and stress, why wouldn't he be? "I just need to do my things and do them well and see if that's gonna be good enough."

Tiger in *lilac* had given the people what they wanted, namely superlative play that led to birdies and one or two muted fist pumps. Afterward, he answered journalists' questions by the mammoth, ancient water oak by the clubhouse—The Tree—not in the club's swanky new Press Center. He said something slightly humorous about the next day's early start time. The media asked him . . . something. Tiger said . . . something. Truth is, we've heard this man interviewed so many times and he's usually so bland that I think we tune out his words and just watch for emotion on that extraordinary face and listen to his diction:

short phrases punctuated by long stops and rising inflection—uptalking. In his hilarious send-up, comedian Conor Moore has his Tiger sniff, pull the neck on his red shirt, cough, look away, and observe that "it's really tough out there."

History does not record what Woods did that night in his gorgeous rental house between the wide brown Savannah River and a golf course. At some point he might have raised a glass to the fine people in the Texas Back Institute Center for Disc Replacement. One more day, vertebrae!

Koepka shared his thoughts at the media center. He is such a gust of fresh air, a great golfer who seems to embrace the art as much as the science of the greatest game. He plays fast, is unhappy with those who don't, and has a firm policy against bitching about course conditions or the weather. He seemed genuinely confused or amused by the nerdy questions he was getting, and he continued to sound like a sage. We could, maybe should, embroider these phrases on golf towels. Here's more wisdom from Kafka. Koepka.

"I've been playing this game, twenty-two, twenty-three years; nothing's going to change overnight.

"I know how to play the game. I just know how to hit the ball.

"I'm just gonna go out and do what I normally do.

"Just gonna tee it up, look where I wanna hit it, and fire at it."

PART FOUR

The Back Nine on Sunday

"Chills. *Chills.*"

—Ryan Gunnels, sixteen, a junior at Richmond Academy in Augusta, on what he felt as he stood by the eighteenth green in the final moments of the 2019 Masters

Sunday, April 14

9:09 am	Koepka	66-71-69=	-10	4
9:20	Finau	70-71-64=	-11	T-2
9:20	Woods	70-68-67=	-11	T-2
9:20	Molinari	70-67-66=	-13	1

Booths filled fast at the Waffle House by the Bobby Jones Expressway. Patrons read their phones, scanned plastic menus, expressed golf-related opinions, and wondered if anyone had had the goddamn sense to bring a canteen of Bloody Marys. Waitresses said "Whatcha have, hon?" and relayed the orders in a slightly raised voice for the cook, whose back was to the room and who scraped and chopped a metal spatula on the sizzling grill as if he had eight arms, like Vishnu. The diners could and did request hash browns scattered, covered, smothered, chunked, topped, or peppered; Yankee boys ate grits because when in Rome; they drank gallons of coffee; they tipped exorbitantly; and then they were gone, for the crazy early start of the fourth round of the 2019 Masters. Balls in the air at seven-thirty! It made for an early morning after the night before.

No one saw the dawning sun rise at 6:59, just lightening shades of gray beaming into a cool morning. It would be a pleasant day to play or to spectate, no jacket required. About seventy-two degrees.

Tiger had been up well before the grit-munching waffle eaters, having put his feet on the floor at a quarter to four. An early morning tee time was a major inconvenience for a guy whose stiff, achy body took a long while to get limber enough to even start warming up. But with bad weather forecast for late afternoon, the pro-active Augusta National and Masters authorities decreed the early start, with play in threesomes instead of pairs, and half the field beginning their rounds on ten and half on one. All of it was unprecedented.

In the dim gray light players rolled their courtesy cars slowly up the deep green tunnel of Magnolia Lane. They were all dark gray Mercedes-Benz SUVs except for two: Tiger had a black one and Ricky Fowler drove a green Maybach. Some participants would roll back in a year in another luxury car, but others might never see this place again.

Patrons streaming in from another corner of the property were excited to the point of nervousness, but also exhilarated by portent and promise. Tiger felt pressure, too, he said, and that he always did. But it was a familiar process he knew and accepted as part of the experience. Recognizing, if not exactly embracing the high stress of big moments, he didn't have to struggle to control a suddenly jumpy and disorganized brain because, he said, his senses sharpened as the competition reached its climax. He got more focused, not less.

Some say that the greatest golf tournament ever played was great in part because the three top contenders symbolized eras as well as themselves. Past, present, and future collided in the 1960 US Open at Cherry Hills in the persons of Hogan, Palmer, and Nicklaus. The present won, by the way. The divisions were less sharp in the 2019 Masters, however. Although Koepka and Molinari were most emphatically key players in the here and now at the very top of professional golf and Finau looked poised to join them in a major winner's circle soon, Tiger refused to play the Ghost of Christmas Past. They say time is an athlete's real enemy, not the other players, but the forty-three-year-old Woods was not giving in to the ticking clock. At least not yet.

They were four genius golfers playing at full genius levels. How were they different? How were they the same?

In a most superficial way, they were indistinguishable, in that the Cablanasian, the Polynesian, the Italian, and the generic, plain-vanilla Koepka all arrived on the first tee in the same brand of clothing. How embarrassing! But the four at least all sported a clean look, because Nike endorsers wear only the swoosh and no competing logos— as opposed to the six, eight, or ten disparate sales messages on some other golfers' bodies. The clear, uncluttered signage would be worth many millions this day to the giant marketer. When Woods contended in the 2018 Valspar, a mere regular tour event, CNBC business reporter Dominic Chu estimated the "brand exposure" from TV and online was worth $10.8 million to Nike. With four leading men wearing the swoosh, and it being the Masters, the value to the brand was astronomical.

In the game of books and covers, Finau was a mid-major small forward; Molinari was a pocket square and a tailored gray suit away from being the CEO of Armani or Ferrari; and Koepka was the all-star leftfielder who hits with power to all fields. Given what we know, it's hard not to picture alternate reality Tiger looking lethal in dark clothes, wraparound shades, and a tactical gun belt.

Best athlete? Finau, probably, because he excelled in the run, jump, catch, and throw of basketball, a sport in which he was recruited to play collegiately. He can stand flat-footed under a hoop and dunk. Molinari skis and snowboards. Koepka at least *looks* like a jock. He comes from a baseball family and played as a kid; they still take a knee in Pittsburgh at the mention of Brooks's great uncle, former Pirates shortstop Dick Groat. Tiger's only games outside golf were not sports and required only a couch and a controller, except for scuba diving and ping-pong during Ryder Cups.

Masters records: with his four wins and nine other finishes in the top ten, Tiger's accomplishments in Augusta dwarfed that of the other three. In three tries, Koepka's best result was a T-11 in '17 (he hadn't played in '18 due to a wrist injury). Moli's highwater mark in seven Masters had been a T-20; he'd missed the cut twice and hadn't even been invited to the party in '15 and '16. As mentioned, Finau was almost a blank slate, having only played the tournament once before.

Kids: Tony, four; Tiger, two; Frankie, two; Brooks, on deck. Majors won: Tiger, fourteen; Brooks, four; Frankie, one; Tony, soon come. Confidence, technique, momentum, astrological? All three would rank very high.

Ages: Koepka, twenty-eight; Finau, twenty-nine; Molinari, thirty-six; Woods, forty-three.

They resided in London; Lehi, Utah; and Jupiter, Florida. Molinari cared very deeply about two soccer clubs, West Ham, in England, and Internazionale Milano back in Italy. Finau is a Los Angeles Lakers fan, judging by the hat. Tiger is often seen sitting courtside at Orlando Magic games.

Number of times winning a major when trailing after three rounds: Molinari, one; Koepka, one; Woods, none.

As for fan support, there was no comparison. Just as clapping hands kept Tinker Bell from dying, fourth-round Masters fans would create a wave of emotion for Tiger to surf on. The patron favorite popped some gum into his mouth and the game was on.

"Fore, please!" the man on the tee called out. "Tiger Woods, now drivin'."

• • •

A narrative assembled from the simple tally of birdies and bogies posted on the front nine would convey little sense of the gathering tension. Molinari, for example, seasoned his seven pars with one of each but his was an exciting tour of the first half of the course, epitomized by the way he played the sixth. Downhill par threes often feel like breathers but the steeply sloped green on six at Augusta National looks totally uninviting, as if the golfer were being asked to hit and hold an Alp or an Ande. Shots short of the flagstick invited three-putts and balls over it were dead. Francesco went long.

Figurative death would toll if he didn't play his next one exactly right. A little long or short with his pitch and double bogey and a lead change would be in play but Molinari contrived a shot that crawled up the bank on little cat's feet and a putt from about six feet that rolled at such perfect speed and on such a perfect path that the ball didn't touch the sides of the hole when it went in. It was his forty-ninth hole in a row of par or better, one away from the all-time Masters record, and a couple of no-bogies past Ben Hogan. His short game was superb; his hands on a putter looked perfectly relaxed yet totally in control, like Federer with a tennis racquet or Clapton with a guitar. Moli led the field by three.

And then he led by one, because on seven, Tiger spun one

to within a few inches for birdie three, while Francesco hooked his tee ball and had some pine tree trouble. He punched his ball back into play, leaving a short but awkward pitch. But then the hill on the far side of the hole didn't help like it was supposed to, the putt from two yards didn't break the way it was supposed to, and Molinari earned his first bogey since Thursday afternoon, on the eleventh hole. He'd been nineteen for nineteen at making pars after missing greens.

While Francesco scrambled and recovered over and over, his opponent in a red shirt was in the midst of an old timey shot-maker/ball-striker round in the mode of Trevino or Hogan. With his driver sliding right here and a drawing left there, and judicious shots to greens punctuated by spectacular ones such as that sweet one into seven, Tiger seemed to be in full control, although he could not poke his nose out front. His eerily calm concentration reminded some of the great mentalist, Nicklaus.

With birdies on seven and eight and a par on nine, Woods would shoot a one-under thirty-five.

A hole ahead of the Tiger-Tony-Frankie group, Koepka played and walked with his usual air of invincibility. The safecracker with muscles went for every pin, eschewing all opportunities to play it safe. He also birdied the eighth, the hardest of the Augusta National par fives. He shot the front nine in one-under, matching Woods.

The only non-major winner in the final pairing looked unfazed by it all but he didn't look like we'd expected; Finau had almost promised to wear a shirt to match the coveted jacket but here he was in a plain white polo.

"I wear green on Sunday because it's my mom's favorite color, but green goes pretty well Sunday at the Masters, too," he'd said back in the day, when playing and contending in the tournament was only a dream. Honoring Ravena became vital in the wake of her death in a car accident in 2011. Tony missed his mother desperately. Back then, what with mourning her, the demands of his profession—he failed to qualify for the tour five times—and a wife and an eventual family to support, the poor man worried himself into a gastric ulcer. He couldn't walk for five weeks or play golf for eight.

So: no green shirt, but Finau did carry a talisman in his bag—or, rather, his caddie, Greg Bodine, did: an Augusta National logo ball signed by 1971 champ Billy Casper, a good friend, recently deceased, and the only Mormon to have won the Masters—up to now.

The standings after nine holes:

Molinari	-13
Woods	-12
Finau	-11
Koepka	-11

The wind freshened.

And the game changed. Since ugly clicking digital

scoreboards do not litter the greensward at the National, players sometimes must intuit their relative positions via sonar and echolocation. Like bats. On the several holes where none of the old hand-cranked Masters leaderboards were visible, dramatic change was signaled by people yelling very damn loud in nearby arenas. Is that a birdie roar or an eagle roar? A Tiger roar or an Ian Poulter?

"The Masters doesn't begin until the back nine on Sunday" contains enough truth to be endlessly repeated, but if tournament and club co-founder Bobby Jones had had his way, no one would use that phrase, ever. For the immortal Bobby thought "back side" and "back nine" was rather too close to a veiled reference to a human backside. A little Ned Flanders, that. Prissy, but that's the way the Grand Slam winner rolled.

Permission to re-phrase, sir? "The Masters commences in earnest on the inward half of the final round."

Which is wonderful because Augusta National's inward half is the greatest stretch run in sports. Better than the clubhouse turn at Churchill Downs, better than the last quarter mile of the Iditarod, and better than the last lap at Indy, which is identical to the first lap.

The inward half at Augusta National is like nine Fenway Parks: lovely self-contained spaces, each with its own fans, acoustics, and concession stands.

The first Fenway is the tenth hole, with a tee shot so inviting it may make your eyelids tighten. Behind the golfer, as he prepares to launch from this tee, are the practice green, the green and white umbrellas on the veranda, the Oak, and the clubhouse. To his left are various bright white, immaculately landscaped, black-shuttered "cottages," an understatement on the order of saying that Lake Erie is a pond. Out in front: immensity.

You hit off a cliff. There's a 175-foot drop from the tee on ten to the bridge over the creek on twelve; it would be fun for us patrons to ski the ten-to-twelve run this winter if they get some snow. Maybe they could put in a rope tow? Something for the suggestion box.

But seriously: if you can swat out a high hook you're in business on ten and you'll have an extra-long time to savor your good shot, as the ball seems to hang in the air there forever. But the golfer whose anti-hook gene prevents a useful curveball is playing for bogey, which was exactly the fate of Tiger and Tony in the final round. Koepka got it up and down from the right bunker with two terrific shots. Molinari made a cold-blooded green-in-regulation, two-putt par, and now led by two.

Finau missed his six-foot putt for par on ten, but at least he'd done so with dispatch and without resorting to the singularly annoying habit of many modern pro golfers, a pre-putt study of a topographical map. Green maps are not allowed at the Masters. Players and caddies are not even permitted to make their own. Thank you, Augusta National.

From the tee to the fairway, the eleventh is another

friendly Fenway, more cozy and defined than it used to be, thanks to aggressive planting of evergreens in recent decades. For the second consecutive day, Tiger blew it right of Rush Limbaugh, but for the second consecutive day he had a fairly straightforward shot through the trees. Racing luck.

"I was five feet from him for that shot," recalled local teen Ryan Gunnels. "He was just talking numbers with Joe, but Tiger makes all the decisions. He's the most focused guy out there. It's almost like he's not human or he's in a different world from us."

For Jay Beach, seventeen, Ryan's pal and fellow Tiger partisan, watching the man in black and red all day was equal parts war whoops and stress: "My nerves . . . I was really nervous all day. His putts seemed to take like twenty seconds to get to the hole." The two friends eventually walked up the ski hill to the eighteenth green to watch the finish.

Molinari missed the eleventh fairway by only a couple of yards, but his penalty was much greater than Tiger's. Because of tree branches and angles, he had to hit his second shot low, aim it at the water hazard on the left, and spin it back to the right. Which he did. Ice water. *Sangue freddo.*

The standings after eleven holes:

Molinari	-13
Woods	-11
Koepka	-11
Finau	-10

Then some stuff happened. The standings after twelve holes:

Molinari	-11
Woods	-11
Schauffele	-11
Day	-10
Watson	-10
Koepka	-9
Finau	-8

What stuff? You probably remember: within a few minutes, with the Masters on the line, four of six of the best players in the world hit their damn balls in the creek, from 158 yards. Each man with a water ball scored double bogey five on twelve.

The pin was located far right. The hourglass-shaped green is canted to the right and a flagstick there is a couple of steps farther away than it looks. It was an enticing target, partly because the back bunker and the one by the water were not in your line if you went right at the stick. But with so little room for a ball out there, and the penalty for a miscalculation so severe, who would be bold enough or reckless enough to fire right at the yellow flag?

"Augusta babies know *from the cradle* that you don't shoot at the Sunday pin on twelve," observed former Augusta baby Tim Wright.

Tim should have told Koepka, who went directly at the stick, with a nine iron. For a long couple of seconds, Brooks's Titleist ProV1x hung in the air like a punted football. Mysterious, undetectable winds aloft subtly lowered its apogee and retarded its velocity, forcing the pill to earth three yards short of its goal; the ball rolled backward off the lush green bank and into Rae's Creek. The crowd groaned, loud enough for the threesome coming down eleven to hear. Was that a Koepka groan or a Webb Simpson moan? After his requisite period of fussing and frowning on the twelfth tee, Ian Poulter lofted his wayward ball into the hazard, too.

"I knew it [the wind] was slightly in then all of a sudden it was down," Brooks said later. "We all know on that hole the wind direction changes by the second. It's just a guessing game. Once [the ball] gets above those trees . . ."

Although it looked like he had his hands full on eleven, Tiger was watching.

"Joe and I had noticed Brooksie and Poults were both in the water," Tiger told Henni. "I know from playing with Brooksie a lot that he's got a much stronger ball flight than I do. It pierces through the wind. And for him to come up short? I kind of earmarked [that]."

Furthermore, the ripples on the surface of the pond on eleven indicated a bit of wind against and from the left. From this data and the washed balls of his fellow competitors, Tiger concluded that there was a headwind on twelve that could not be felt on the face or detected from tossing up leaves of grass.

Missed putts and doubles for Koepka and Poulter, with Ian and Webb Simpson enacting a slow-moving drama that gave the three on the tee more time to think and to worry. In hell, they make you watch Webb Simpson putt.

The coast finally cleared. The creek, the bunkers, and the green on twelve present a simple, harmonious tableau of shapes and colors. Someone non-literal should paint it, a Japanese landscape artist, perhaps. Maybe a modern-day Francisco Goya could bring out the hole's evil beauty.

Moli looked up; no wind vexed the treetops, but he knew it was up there. He decided to take an extra club—an eight— but to hold something back; an inch of grip protruded above his hands. He was trying to contrive a lower shot that might be less affected by the mysterious, swirling wind, but, just like Brooksie and Poults, he took dead aim at the inviting pin, and like them, he came up short. His Callaway ball with two red dots crawled down the steep creek bank and into the drink.

Embedded within the subsequent group gasp were sounds indicating what was in the heart of many hearts, that this shocking failure by the machine-like Moli was good for Tiger. But cheering a mistake is not done in golf; it's especially not done at the Masters, where such behavior can get the offending patron escorted off the grounds by a man with a gun. Mr. Jones felt very strongly about this. Golf stands in opposition to the dubious sportsmanship in tennis, in which opponents celebrate each other's double-faults and mishits with a pump of the fist.

But you can exclaim about anything you want if you're just reacting to the scoreboard. The board watchers arrayed around the eighteenth green screamed as one when the operator took down Francesco's red 13 and replaced it with an 11. "The crowd went crazy," remembered Jay Beach. "Everyone on eighteen was going insane."

Tiger's turn on twelve. His blank face showed a man in full cold mode. Gathering data even as he took his stance, he aimed a nine iron thirty feet left of the stick and hooked it a little just be sure; the ball cleared the front bunker and stopped short of the back bunker and the patrons cheered.

Tony now. He searched the area for clues on wind direction and speed, chose a club, and aimed at Tiger's ball. "I was going to hit a fade, and there was a puff of wind from the left," Finau recalled. The Utahn's ball soared even higher than Koepka's, but, like a turkey vulture, it was majestic in flight and ugly on the ground. It, too, landed on the lush green bank and fell back into the creek. "He hit it flush, but you could see it just get killed at its peak," Tiger said.

Geez, Tony, I asked: after those other three came up short, why didn't you . . . ? Finau explained that virtually in the middle of his punchy, three-quarter swing, he'd sensed that he was aimed too far left, so he adjusted microscopically to the right. To his great regret.

Cunning had defeated daring.

Incredulity reigned. With three of the leaders up the creek, the atmosphere felt crazy and unsettled. Who was in, who was out, and most of all, for most people, where was Tiger?

"I was by those stands by thirteen green and fourteen tee," recalled Gilbert Freeman, the Dallas golf pro. "If you're in just the right spot and you have binoculars, you can see way back to the twelfth green, but you can't see the tee. We heard the disappointed groans when someone—two some-ones—hit it in the water. Apparently, the third guy was safe. The safe guy would be revealed by who walked up on the green first. 'It's Tiger!' a couple of the binocular guys said, and that crowd went nuts.

"It was like we were a collective One, all of us pulling for the same thing."

What an opera: Spotting three maintenance men watching from the azalea bushes, and observing miscella-neous organic schmutz in his line, Tiger requested they bring down their leaf blowers and clear his path to the hole. They did. Moli missed from ten: double bogey. Tiger holed from six for a two-putt par. Finau missed from five and posted a double, too. Light rain began to fall. Umbrellas opened like azaleas blooming.

On the thirteenth tee, with the surge of adrenaline only a double bogey can provide—a condition known colloqui-ally as red ass—Koepka blasted his drive over the trees and around the corner and had only an eight-iron left to the green on the par five.

"I wasn't deflated," Finau recalled in our chat during his

pro-am round at Colonial a month later. "I knew I'd get eagle and birdie looks on the final six holes. But I also knew I'd have to play perfectly."

Woods would describe the new situation as "Pandora's box, now opened up . . . Fast forward to thirteen. Brooksie makes eagle. I make birdie. Finau makes birdie. Cantlay . . . DJ's making a run, Bubba just got to ten-under quickly. Four guys are tied for the lead (at eleven-under). Now seven guys have a legitimate chance to win with six holes to go."

Then the subtle game within the endgame began, the process of memorizing scoreboards and listening for mighty blasts of sound.

"It got very interesting trying to figure it all out," Tiger told Henni. He studied the leaderboard on thirteen as if there'd be a test. "I wanted to see where they all were, what holes they were on, in case I hear any roars. Who that might be. I wanna know."

The rain eased up. The tournament heated up.

Patrick Cantlay grabbed the lead at -12 after an eagle on fifteen but he was running out of holes. Schauffele joined him at twelve under. Then it was Schauffele alone. Then Xander got company. The racecars charged to the finish line, bumping doors, trading paint. After fourteen holes, we had, approximately:

Woods, Molinari, Schauffele   -12
Koepka, DJ, Day, Cantlay (?)   -11

Then DJ birdied seventeen, causing a four-way tie at the top at -12. Then Koepka's eagle putt on fifteen *just* missed, and with his resultant birdie four, there was a *five*-way tie.

Tony 'n' Tiger blasted long, straight drives on fifteen and both hit the green with ease in two with irons and would have two-putt birdies in a minute, but before that Moli misplayed three consecutive shots, which cost him big. He drove slightly right into the orange straw beneath the pines and could not go for the green in two. He chipped out but too firmly, his ball running through the fairway at the bottom of the hill by about a step into the left rough, on ragged ground that had been stepped on by many patrons' feet.

There are three tough shots on the inward half, Patrick Reed had told us: the tee balls on twelve and eighteen, and this, the pitch up to the fifteenth green.

Then the worst happened: Molinari lost control of the height of the wedge shot, and his ball flew way the hell up into a pine tree that shouldn't have been in play. The Callaway ball clipped a branch and fell into the middle of the pond with a sad splash. Cheers erupted when the placards were changed on the scoreboards on seventeen and eighteen—a red 13 for Tiger, and the lead alone; a red 10 for Signor Francesco.

On sixteen, as Koepka watched from seventeen, Tiger hit an eight iron with a little draw and his Bridgestone ball caught the slope just right; it was another in a series of terrific iron shots, this one a sort-of re-creation of that impossible slow-mo chip from 2005. The 2019 version didn't go in, but almost, and Woods had a kick-in to go to fourteen under, and the lead by two. Didn't he?

Tiger told Henni: "I hit it close on sixteen so as I'm leaving sixteen tee, I take one last look at the board. 'If I make birdie here and get to fourteen-under, how many guys have a chance to get to fourteen—if I make par the last two holes.'

"Like any other sport you want to know time and distance."

There were two more random-seeming cheers from far away; they were the aftershocks from the scoreboard crowds reacting to Tiger's two on sixteen.

In the din on the short walk to the seventeenth tee, while people all around him were losing their heads, Tiger kept his. His unconscious brain searched for useful precedent and found it. It was 2005 again: fourteen years before, after he'd shocked the world by surging ahead by two with his chip-in birdie on sixteen, euphoria or something fogged his execution and he'd finished, shockingly, with two bogies, and was pretty lucky to have beaten Chris DiMarco.

The tournament leader resolved not to let that happen again; he resolved so hard with his tee ball that it looked like he might crack the head on his M5. It was a slider, perfectly struck and flawlessly controlled, and way the eff out there.

Up ahead, the World Number One kept firing at it. Koepka's super-aggressive style fit the moment and gave crystal clear insight into who this guy is as a competitor:

Brooks is out there for a win, not a high finish. He hit good to great irons on every hole on the inward half except for a so-so shot on sixteen, but had buzzard's luck with his Scotty Cameron T10 Select Newport 2 on the marble-hard greens. He'd made that eight-foot eagle putt on thirteen but otherwise . . . Putts grazed lips. They refused to come in. They walked on by. On eighteen, from 123 yards out, he hit it close one last time.

With the same up-tempo slash he'd just used with the driver, Tiger hit a forceful cut at the flag on seventeen from 143 yards, which hit and stuck, and Our Guy was home free. Probably. After a cautious two-putt he heard rapturous emanations from his gallery, but gave no indication that he was leaving his private concentration zone. Was he still time traveling, still back in '05? He didn't say.

Up at the green, Ryan Gunnels and Jay Beach had by this time wiggled and hopped into greenside seats, finding themselves next to a willowy woman in a green jacket: former Secretary of State Condoleezza Rice. They chatted. "I asked her kinda what it's like being one of the only girl members," recalled Ryan.

As the hyperventilating gallery grew as quiet as it could get, Woods stood behind his ball on the eighteenth tee with a three-wood in his hands. He immersed himself mentally in the challenge of the moment. He removed the inhibition of fear. He harnessed self-belief and discipline. And then he swung. Hard.

As Patrick Reed had said, the tee shot on eighteen puts the

lie to the idea that Augusta National is a wide-open course, but Tiger's low, smashed slider stayed inside the corridor of trees. The ball rolled right, however, according to its spin, leaving an awkward second shot that would become pretty damn hard if Koepka made his eight-foot putt for birdie to get within one.

One difficulty of recalling the next few minutes—or all the minutes in the 2019 Masters—is that the reader knows how the drama turned out. But live, in the moment, nothing was inevitable. Koepka had yet another birdie putt inside ten feet and making it was going to change everything.

CBS-TV reporter Amanda Balionis debriefed Brooks a couple of minutes later. Tell us about eighteen, she said.

"Don't know if I can say it on the air," replied Golf Yoda. A good putt he'd hit. In the ball didn't go.

Now a bogey five would earn Tiger a win by one over Brooks, Xander, and DJ. The smart move would be to use all five shots. He did. From the right edge of the fairway, with tree limbs impinging on his line, and 169 yards left to the hole, Tiger aimed way left and spun the ball back to the right. He'd cleverly left a forty yard third that would not have to traverse any pits of bright white powdered quartz. This was very close to the way Hogan played the hole when he had a bogey to win in 1951.

On the other hand: in a similar situation in 1961, tournament leader Arnold Palmer, needing a par to win, shook patrons' hands and accepted patrons' pats on the back as he walked up the ultimate fairway—then contrived to lose by one after scoring a double bogey. That would not be Tiger's fate; he continued to wear his game face and apart from taking his hat off for a moment, he did not acknowledge the cheers. On TV, Billy Kratzert delivered more of his characteristic verbless sentences. "The determination to come back," he said. "To have this opportunity."

Tiger two-putted from ten feet. Two years after back problems almost crippled him, a decade after a devastating domestic scandal, eleven years since winning his last major, and fourteen years removed from his last first in the Masters—he'd won again. He threw his head back and roared. All happy hell broke loose.

Tiger hugged Tony, shook the hands of Tony's caddie and of Moli and Moli's caddie, then delightedly hugged the third loyal looper in the group, his man, Joe LaCava. Then came home-from-the-war embraces of his son, his mother, his daughter, and his girlfriend. There followed four more whooping hugs with other intimates, then a big one for Steinie.

Suddenly: chanting! "Ti-ger, Ti-ger, Ti-ger"—there were ten reps, and a few more later; it was an honor never bestowed on even the greatest Masters heroes, Jack and Arnie, although it should be said that people chant more now than they used to.

As if he were a speedboat and his mom and kids and girlfriend were attached water skiers, the new champ led the way on a brisk uphill walk to the clubhouse. Giddy fans reached out for a touch from the old/new Master.

Waiting for him outside the scoring area were some of his brother golf pros. Tiger laughed with and clasped the right hands of Trevor Immelman, Zach Johnson, Ricky Fowler, Justin Thomas, Bubba Watson, Ian Poulter, Xander Schauffele, and Bernhard Langer. Then, standing apart from the others was the first among equals, Koepka. They hugged.

"You finish second place, you're a little bummed out," Brooks told the press later, but he wasn't bummed out this time, he said, and he knew he wasn't alone. "After he won there on eighteen there was just a monsoon of people. It's incredible."

A *monsoon* of people.

As TV showed replays of Tiger embracing Earl way back when, and Tiger with armfuls of his own kids just now, Jim Nantz said, "The completion of one of the great comebacks in any sport, all-time," and then Jim and Tiger were hustling to the studio in the Butler Cabin for part one of the Presentation of the Threads. Part two of the green jacket ceremony was the real deal, in which people would be thanked and speeches made. It would take place on the putting green after the brief interlude on TV.

Ms. Balionis caught up with Francesco. "I think I made a few new fans today with those two double bogies," he said with a rueful smile. "On twelve: just a bad swing. Fifteen, I just made a mess.

"I'm proud of the way I stayed calm even after making

mistakes . . . On the back nine just a couple of instances where I wasn't aggressive and kind of lost focus a little bit which is weird to say in these conditions but it's been a long week and it's not easy to hit every shot one hundred percent."

Presently the man who *did* seem to hit every shot one hundred percent had taken a seat in the Butler Cabin's cool basement. Across from him were Chairman Ridley and Nantz. To his left sat Patrick Reed, who wore a green jacket and was holding another one. To his right was Viktor Hovland, the low amateur in the competition. When it was his turn to say a few words, the smiling young man from Oslo gave maximum credit to his Oklahoma State University golf coach, Alan Bratton, who had caddied for him.

In response to Nantz, Tiger attempted to describe how and why he'd had about one shot's worth more mental endurance than the others. He'd stayed present and focused and had kept control of his emotions, he said, but mostly he was "just trying to plod my way around the golf course all day, just plod my way around. All of a sudden I had the lead"—an apt reminder of the Immortal Meltdown on Twelve.

There is a call and response tradition in sports in which a reporter asks the new champ of anything, "Has it sunk in yet?" and the new champ is virtually required to say "no." Nantz didn't bother with this but Henni and Tiger saluted the ritual in the very first exchange in their interview.

But I say sinking in isn't worth all that much. Sinking in

is for retirement years and gazing at the fire. Sinking in is for the jeweler's chisel on the trophy. Maybe Tiger should stay in the present as much as possible regarding the 2019 Masters, to keep his glorious lucky comeback win top-of-mind as long as he can, to never just file it away. For if ever there was a moment to savor, this was it.

"To have my kids there," Tiger said to Fred, Jim, Viktor, Patrick, and the millions watching at home. "It's come full circle. My dad was here in '97. Now I'm the dad."

With that, Reed rose, Tiger got to his feet, and the others stood back. The defending champ held out the jacket and the new champ found the arm holes.

"It fits!" Tiger said.

Roars Echo

~

Six weeks after the Masters, Jack Nicklaus had his own tournament with its own coat, a gray one. The Memorial Tournament presented by Nationwide is played on Muirfield Village Golf Club, arguably the best course on the tour not named Augusta National, so when Jack comes into the CBS-TV booth to say a few words, the conversation is often of the course itself. With the death of co-designer Desmond Muirhead in 2002, it's left to Nicklaus to describe their creation of a magnificent playground from mere farmland.

But this year, the Memorial talk was of Tiger. And Jack was the man to talk to about this, too, because Tiger's lifelong obsession had become a media and fan obsession: equaling or passing the Nicklaus record of eighteen major wins. Jack had won six green jackets; now Tiger had five.

The happy glow around Woods had persisted as if there was radium in his gum. Man, did he bring the people out;

he was playing this week in suburban Columbus, Ohio, for which Jack was grateful.

"He should concentrate on what *he* has to do," to reach eighteen, Jack said. "And only play when he's one hundred percent physically, and mentally as well. He has ten-plus more years of [major] championships and he could win one a year . . ."

Tiger walked onto a tee and gazed at his target. "He's a different person," said the tournament host in voice-over. "Very relaxed. He used to play with high energy, but he doesn't do that now. He used to be hi-bye but now you can actually have a conversation with him."

Later, the cameras found Tiger in the aftermath of making a double bogey on a par five; he didn't seem to be taking it too hard. "[In the past,] he wouldn't have been laughing and smiling after a seven," Jack said. "It's a different personality."

In the Men's Grille at Augusta Country Club, where the arbiters of the game and the game of life reside, opinions are mixed regarding a rebooted Tiger. We should recall that when Tigermania hit town in '97, impolite Yankee hordes arrived with him, and a well-liked local man lost his life trying to supply their badges. Also, this slice of Augusta is as conservative as a blue suit; the Woods marital mess did not play well here. Some in the room dislike his screaming, fist pumping self-congratulation when he wins. Or his swearing when shots go awry.

"I'll give him six months to see if he screws up again," says one of the ACC commentators.

Jerry Matheis, who is in wealth management, provided the countervailing opinion: "The amount of affection he showed to his kids and his mom changed a lot of minds around here."

Their golf pro holds a nuanced view of the fall and rise of Tiger Woods. "First," says Tommy Brannen, "his agent must be really good. Steinberg? The way he handled the reconstruction of who [Tiger] is, his re-emergence as a person—that's impressive.

"The millennials all love Tiger while the racist generation still has its doubts. But show me one guy who didn't get a tear [in his eye] when his family surrounded him after he won.

"I see the Earl coming out in him physically, but his mind might be as sharp as it's ever been."

Brannen and Nicklaus have summed up two confusing aspects of this intriguing man. It was regarded as a one-off miracle when Jack won the Masters at age forty-six, but the Bear foresees Tiger winning or threatening to win majors for another decade, until age fifty-three. And Tommy and others, noticing Woods's resolutely stoic in-game look last April, detect actual improvement in his attitude as a competitor. Tiger didn't seem to be tamping down emotional surges so much as not even having them.

As he tapped in for the win, Tiger tapped into our intense and undying interest in tales of redemption. His story is irresistible: he fell from such a high place that he was halfway to earth before we mere mortals even recognized him as one of us. The triumphant public Tiger had been a compelling figure, winning golf championships with apparent ease while endorsing iconic brands in his spare time. But the private Tiger was out of reach, so protected, sequestered, and remote that he was more symbol than person. His public misadventure was as spectacular as his victories had been and was excruciating to watch. But impossible not to watch, because it was on Letterman and Leno and in the paper, and not just the *Enquirer*.

He became the butt of jokes, then an object of pity. But, maybe, the higher the fall, the bigger the bounce. When Tiger's trials segued from the ethical arena into physical agony requiring multiple surgeries and endless, exhausting rehab, the machinery of public sympathy re-engaged. It was much easier to pull for someone recovering from grievous injury than it was a serial philanderer.

Before the fall, we loved and marveled at what he accomplished so much that we forgave his disregard for the pleasantries of human interaction, like kindness and simple politeness. But then the window opened. When we saw a private world that gave the finger to golf's culture of honor and ethical comportment, the reaction was fierce, if sometimes a bit holier-than-thou.

The champion's return to the top proceeded on two fronts: the slow, steady resurrection of his public image, and his determined battle against injuries that would have ended the career of a lesser man. He will have us glued to the tube and chanting his name for years to come.

Or:

Age could lead to shorter hitting and weakened vision and trouble with short putts. Arthritis—which everyone gets a little or a lot of as they age—could make for a creakier swing and less tolerance for practice. His fused spine might cause overload on the nearby discs, leading to declining stability and flexibility and something painful called adjacent segment disease.

Time will reveal which it will be. But even if this amazing performer has only one or two more good years—or none, or ten—at least we had the 2019 Masters. At least we had that moment.

So, thanks, Tiger. Thanks for roaring back.

The Whole World Turned Into the 2019 Masters

The next few months posed but didn't fully answer several questions regarding the wondrous life of Tiger Woods.

What he'd do for an encore was question one, of course. Woods had three more majors to play following his thrilling win in Augusta. Might he defy the odds and his age one more time and pluck another win from the hands of Koepka, Molinari, Finau, and company? While the interest in Tiger never wanes, his crowds now seemed bigger, more adhesive, and more adoring than ever. He was a hero, a paragon renewed, and not merely a golfer people liked.

In professional golf's re-jiggered schedule, the PGA Championship is the next big one after the Masters. This year the host was Bethpage Black, the fearsome municipal track out on Long Island. To feel a touch of home during the week, Tiger docked his yacht at the Oyster Bay Marine Center, about thirteen miles from the first tee. "Privacy," a 90-footer with a crew of nine, contains a gym, a theater, white carpet, white silk walls, possibly a jai alai court, and definitely 6,500 square feet. Sleeping there would allow Tiger to avoid the notoriously thick car traffic in the area, plus he'd save the cost of a room at Extended Stay America in Melville or wherever. On the other hand, the marina charged a fee of over $1,000 a day.

Tiger had focused on picking the kids up from school and taking them to soccer practice in the thirty-two days between the Masters and the PGA. He played in no tournaments during that time. It showed; he looked tired and creaky at Bethpage and he couldn't hit a fairway. His 72-73 missed the cut by one. Koepka, on the other hand, combining long, straight hitting with impeccable putting, seemed in the bloom of youth. Brooksie opened with 63-65—a 36-hole record in a major—on his way to a two-stroke win over Dustin Johnson, who had shared runner-up status with Koepka at Augusta.

"Just wasn't moving the way I needed to," Tiger told the media on Friday afternoon, May 17. "That's the way it goes. There's going to be days and weeks where it's just not going to work, and today was one of those days."

Next up on May 30 was Jack's tournament, the Memorial, at Muirfield Village Golf Club in Dublin, Ohio. With a flurry of birdies in the final round, Tiger finished tied for ninth place, ten shots behind the winner, Patrick Cantlay. Woods was animated in his post-round interview with Henni Zuel, demonstrating his hip turn and body rotation, the kind of thing he never does in the usual media scrum. "It was a good practice week," Tiger said.

After a two-week rest, it was on to the US Open at Pebble Beach, where he had once won by fifteen shots. But his best-ever tournament performance nineteen years earlier now seemed like a distant memory. The cool, sullen mid-June weather bothered him; he mentioned his strong desire for temperatures warmer than the fifty-degree chill that gripped the Monterey Peninsula that week. As those of us over forty well know, cold aggravates our aches apains; KT medical tape peeked out of his shirt and stuck to his sore neck. His crowds were huge and enthusiastic, but they didn't get what they wanted.

With another flurry of almost meaningless birdies on the final nine holes Tiger finished at two-under, eleven shots behind the winner, Gary Woodland, in a seven-way tie for 21st. Two 2019 Masters rivals fared better. Koepka finished second, three shots back; Molinari, tied for 16th.

"I'm going to take a little bit of time off and enjoy some family time," the weary Woods told the press afterwards.

A couple of days later, Tiger, Erica, and the kids were spotted in Bangkok. The photo going around showed all four, post-flight, in matching yellow t-shirts. Out of the frame was Tida, Tiger's mom, who as you may recall is Thai. During the Woods family two-week summer vacation there was no golf club touching. Afterwards they went back to Florida and then on to Europe.

"We had the greatest time," Tiger told the media at his presser before the Open Championship in mid-July. "Sam's birthday was over there. We rode elephants, went on a safari. They understand the culture a little bit more, the things they didn't really know about. It was an experience, especially since my mom's health is diminishing and we're not sure how many times she can do this."

People noticed that Tiger had played no Scottish Open or John Deere Classic to warm up his engine; Padraig Harrington, who is twice an Open champion, wondered aloud about how serious Woods was about winning. But he and we should not forget what a monumental challenge golf tournaments have become for post-surgical, middle-aged Tiger. Recall that his early start time on Sunday at the Masters had required him to hit the deck at 3:45 a.m. in order to get his body and mind ready for the day's challenges.

If Tiger—or anyone—had thought it was cool at Pebble Beach, then the Dunluce Course at Royal Portrush in Northern Ireland was downright frigid. And rainy. Wincing at times and walking and swinging more slowly than in April, Woods's 78-70 missed the cut by five shots. (Finau finished third, eight strokes behind runaway winner Shane Lowry of Ireland; Koepka tied for fourth, concluding his fantastic major season; and Molinari finished tied for eleventh, twelve strokes back.)

"Gonna take a few weeks off and rest up for the playoffs," the Masters champion said.

"I don't have the flexibility I used to have and I never will.

"I have to make certain adaptations.

"I just want some time off, to get away from it.

"I just wanna go home."

Thus, we had our answer to our questions about Acts Two through Four in in the 2019 majors, and a reliable predictor of Tiger's tournament future. There will be fewer of them—probably just the Masters, the Opens, the PGA, and a selection of exalted events that would be blessed by his presence. It was a schedule that had been previewed by that other injured king of comeback, Ben Hogan.

• • •

In the months since the Masters, I'd been wondering about Ms. Zuel, the charming interviewer with GOLFTV. Given my status as Tiger's 120th biographer, I wanted to know why Henni's post-Masters back-and-forth with the new champion was the best, or one of the best interviews Tiger had ever given. Everyone from Oprah to Ed Bradley of *60 Minutes* to Jimmy Roberts had tried and failed to draw him out, and the late, great Dan Jenkins couldn't even get Woods to open his mouth.

The answer to that mystery had been hiding in plain sight since late November 2018. Because I'd rather four-putt than read a press release, I'd missed the one headlined "Tiger Woods and Discovery's GOLFTV Announce Exclusive Long-term Global Content Partnership."

The release went on to reveal that GOLFTV, a

streaming-video service co-owned by Discovery Inc. and the PGA Tour, "will collaborate with Woods on a wide range of programming, content creation, and storytelling opportunities that will offer fans an authentic and regular look into the life, mind and performance of the game's ultimate icon."

And then there are about 500 words quoting the game's ultimate icon saying things he surely didn't say, in a language no one uses except in press releases. If we are to believe this corporate statement, Tiger has been itchin' to get his story out: "I love the vision of GOLFTV and the ambition for it to become the premier destination for golf entertainment worldwide. To have my own platform to communicate is the culmination of a lot of hard work from my team and the team at Discovery . . . I can't wait to share my knowledge."

Tiger giving time to Henni Zuel and giving her his best stuff had therefore merely been the fulfillment of a contractual duty. He'd been paid for it, in other words. Paying sources is anathema in journalism but this deal wouldn't be about fact-checkable reporting so much as entertainment and public relations. What's his pay? Gerry Smith of Bloomberg writes that Tiger will get a cut of subscription revenue. That could be a lot.

And speaking of money: according to the sports marketing experts quoted by Martha C. White in her story at nbcnews.com, Woods's win in April was a financial windfall for a variety of entities. Himself, first of all: "I would not be surprised if, in the long run, this win in Augusta is worth

$50 to $100 million in future benefits to Tiger," said Richard Burton, the David Falk professor of sports management at Syracuse University. "His appearance fees go up. If he is involved in designing golf courses [he is], his fee goes up. His next Nike contract may be worth more."

Nike will probably be pleased to pay. The marketing giant got about $22.5 million in media exposure from its endorser's fourth round alone, which was basically a four-hour commercial for the swoosh. "He's eclipsed what he provided Nike in brand exposure for the four majors last year with just this one major," Eric Smallwood of Apex Marketing Group told Smith. Smallwood estimated $2.3 million of billboard benefit to Rolex—widely circulated photos showed Tiger holding the trophy with one of its watches wrapped around his wrist—and a combined $1 million-worth of airtime for Bridgestone (golf balls) and Monster, the energy drink maker whose green claw-mark logo decorates Tiger's black golf bag.

If everything from his interviews to his shoes must be monetized, then Woods missed a marketing opportunity by not having an alliance with a CBD oil company. Apparently. Rumors were rife that enhanced gum helped Tiger achieve his very even keel at Augusta; I've watched all the tape numerous times and didn't see Tiger get obviously mad even once, or swear, as he usually does. He didn't even mutter after missed putts, and he's a mutterer. CBD oil is as natural as aspirin—whose active ingredient comes from willow tree bark—and my doctor is lately telling me to put a couple of sub-lingual drops in my mouth twice a day, to help with my sore muscles and my unfocused wandering. Some bigtime golf pros endorse the stuff, among them Bubba Watson, Lucas Glover, Scott Piercy, Scott McCarron, and Charley Hoffman. Phil Mickelson, also a notable gum chewer during the Masters, was photographed during the tournament with a dropper in his mouth. Someday CBD oil may be considered as benign and uncontroversial as aspirin, but nowadays it's a tricky bit of business, because the oil comes from the cannabis plant, and cannabis contains a chemical called THC, the psychoactive ingredient in marijuana. Although eleven states and the District of Columbia have legalized recreational use of the weed, Tour players who test positive for THC get suspended, as recently happened with Robert Garrigus.

The situation is in flux. After allowing cannabidiol oil, the Tour flipped in early April, before the Masters. On or about April 2, the bosses sent the players a letter, which said, in part: "CBD products (like all supplements) pose a risk to athletes because they have limited government regulation and may contain THC . . . Taking a poorly labeled supplement that is contaminated with a prohibited substance is NOT a defense to a violation of the Program."

The use of CBD oil for sufferers of certain serious diseases has been legal in Georgia, by the way, since 2015. So is its in-state production and sale, as of April 17, 2019 (five days after the Masters), when Governor Brian Kemp, rhymes with hemp, signed House Bill 324.

I'd like to know if Tiger is using the supplement—he won't say—and if he is, where I can get some.

• • •

The solemn, sunlit ceremony in the Rose Garden might have been sublime at another time and under different circumstances. Instead it was a "Do I want this or not?" thing, like a chef's salad that might contain one or two grasshoppers.

It started with a tweet, as things so often do in this golden age of social media. This one employed the *National Enquirer*–style book. Tapping on the keys was our Tweeter-in-Chief: "Spoke to @TigerWoods to congratulate him on the great victory he had in yesterday's @TheMasters, & to inform him that because of his incredible Success & Comeback in Sports (Golf) and, more importantly, LIFE, I will be presenting him with the PRESIDENTIAL MEDAL OF FREEDOM!"

What raised eyebrows and made stomachs churn wasn't the identity of the honoree, for Tiger deserves the recognition, although he probably doesn't need it. The first problem was with the honor-or: Trump is such a thoroughgoing and cheerful cheater on the golf course that Rick Reilly felt compelled to pen *Commander in Cheat*, which is a funny book but also quite chilling. A purist, Trump ain't. Golf is kind of a joke to him and a way to make money.

Second problem: the timing. Up to now, the PMF has been a lifetime achievement award for the other thirty-two sportsmen and women who've won it, but Tiger has been making a mighty effort and taking great pains to continue his career for years to come. So why bestow the nation's highest civilian award so soon? What's the rush? Politicians love to be photographed next to the astronaut or the championship team—that's nothing new—so why couldn't Trump have just invited Woods to the White House for tea and a photo op?

This leads us to the second part of the second problem—motivation. We'd hate to think that there was a business purpose in the awarding of this particular Presidential Medal of Freedom, but there was. For a few years now, Tiger's design company has had a deal in place with Trump's golf course project in Dubai, an alliance Tiger's side has been running away from ever since. "Tiger is not in partnership with Mr. Trump or his organization and stating otherwise is absolutely wrong," said Woods spokesman Glenn Greenspan, splitting hairs in 2017. "Tiger Woods Design's contract is with the developer . . . I can't put it any clearer that Tiger Woods Design does not have an agreement with Mr. Trump."

As you can imagine, Donald J. hasn't been so shy about the fact that Tiger is his partner.

"Why does he get the medal? Well, he does business with Trump," commented Richard Painter, the chief ethics lawyer for the George W. Bush administration, putting it bluntly, as he always does.

This did not come from out of nowhere. "Ever since Tiger Woods arrived on the public stage as a golf phenom at age 21, Donald J. Trump has been cultivating him as a celebrity who could add a sheen to his properties around the globe," explained Annie Karni and Kevin Draper in the *New York Times*. "On Monday, Mr. Trump is set to once again seize Mr. Woods's moment."

The plump geriatric golfer and the trim muscular one live near each other in Florida, they've teed it up together at least three times, and, with all attendant fanfare, Trump named a hostel at Trump Doral the Tiger Woods Villa.

They stood together in brilliant May sunshine, both in blue suits and red ties, with the White House forming an impressive background. Trump gassed on for thirteen and a half minutes; Tiger made do with three. "Just a few weeks ago the world turned into the 2019 Masters," said the president in his introduction. He meant "tuned in" but his teleprompter malaprop held a more interesting meaning.

"The amazing Masters experience I just had a few weeks ago was certainly probably the highlight of what I've accomplished in my life on the golf course, to have had that type of experience and come out on top and win," Tiger said. He spoke without notes. Obviously.

• • •

Readers will close this book but we can't close the book on Tiger, not yet. Although he's been derailed a time or two during his journey, his train seems to have more miles of track, and his final stop is unknown. As it is for all of us.

As a boy he was prepared magnificently for golf accomplishment but negligently for interpersonal encounters. As a man he suffered grievous injury from the intensity of his training and practice but he came back from it. The hot-house of fame made his lack of empathy more noticeable and probably made it worse, but he's come back from that, too. With his grit and his unshakeable conviction, Tiger's been like one of those toy punching bags with a weighted bottom, returning to an upright fighting position no matter how often it's hit or how hard, and we admire that.

Just as the Rose Garden medal ceremony was premature, it's a fool's errand to try to place Eldrick T. Woods in his proper historical context just now. We can, however, confidently place him on the first tee at Augusta National on April 9, 2020. It's going to be expensive to be there with him; it turns out that Masters ticket guru Clyde Pilcher misunderestimated the market when we spoke last summer. Eight months before the first shot is hit, the cost of a $375 badge—the 2019 number—has skyrocketed to $12,000, and the price will surely skyrocket even higher.

The dogwoods and azaleas will be blooming pink, white, and red. The rolling hills will be emerald, the bunker sand blindingly white. The tall long-leaf and loblolly pines will sway in the breeze like dancers. The patrons will hold their breath.

"Fore, please," the starter will say into the hush. "Now drivin': Tiger Woods!"

BIBLIOGRAPHY AND SOURCES

Books

GOLF Magazine's Encyclopedia of Golf 1959.

Haney, Hank, with Jaime Diaz. *The Big Miss.* Three Rivers Press, 2012.

Keteyian, Armen, and Jeff Benedict. *Tiger Woods.* Simon & Schuster, 2018.

Manchester, William. *Goodbye, Darkness.* Dell, 1979.

Sampson, Curt. *Chasing Tiger.* Atria Books, 2002.

Sampson, Curt. *Hogan.* Rutledge Hill Press, 1996.

Sampson, Curt. *The Eternal Summer.* Taylor Publishing, 1992.

Sampson, Curt. *The Masters.* Villard, 1998.

Williams, Steve, with Michael Donaldson. *Out of the Rough.* Viking, 2015.

Articles

Fluff Cowan quote: *Eugene Register-Guard,* 6/10/97

TheNarcissisticLife.com

Skip Alexander: *EvansvilleBoneyard.org*; St Petersburg Times, 11/24/97

Earl Woods obit: the *New York Times* and the *Guardian*

Marcus quote: March 4, 2019 *New Yorker*

"Nice fucking shirt" from *Out of the Rough*

Foley quote *New York Times* 5/10/11

120 extra maritals per *Tiger Woods*

Tiger surgeries per *PGA.com*

"How Tiger Woods Won the Back Surgery Lottery" by Gina Kolata *New York Times* 5/15/19

"Babe Could Play" by Curt Sampson *USGA Golf Journal* Jan-Feb 1991

"It's Almost Miraculous" by Adam Kilgore *Washington Post* April 16, 2019

"Tiger Woods US PGA . . ." by Ewan Murray *The Guardian* 5/18/19

"Who is Tony Finau?" by Lee Benson *Deseret News* 3/31/18

"My Shot: Tony Finau" with Guy Yocom *Golf Digest* 8/1/15

"The 94-year-old Masters champion . . ." by Ewan Murray *The Guardian* 4/2/17

"Tiger Woods Speaks Out . . ." by Ryan Herrington *Golf World* 11/3/17

"The Masters: Augusta's Terrible 10th . . ." by Gary van Sickle *Sports Illustrated Golf+* 4/9/13

Greenentrepreneur.com "Was that CBD . . ." by Brendan Bures 4/22/19

ACKNOWLEDGMENTS

First mention goes to Mark Weinstein and Scott Waxman of *Diversion Books*. Mr. Weinstein is an excellent editor.

I acknowledge the help of many others, particularly John Strawn and Nancy Mancini.

Second place for helpful goes to, ladies first: Donna Archer, Sarah Gow, Maggie Lagle, Nicole McLeod, Victoria Student, Cherie Wright, Henni Zuel.

The gentlemen: Danny Fitzgerald, Tim Wright, Jerry Tarde, John Garrity, Jaime Diaz, Gaylen Groce, Peter Jacobsen, Aaron Wise, J.J. Henry, David Jacobsen, Chip Gow, Tony Finau, Gilbert Freeman, Buddy Alexander, Mike Morrow, Dan Strimple, Mike Wright, Clay Montgomery, Pat Perez, Greg Bodine, Martin Piller, Fabian Gomez, Clay Sampson, Bob West, Don van Natta, Tim Brown, Brooks Koepka, John Sampson, Don M. Wilson III, Jordan Snowie, Jerry Matheis, Clyde Pilcher, John Crow Miller, Brad Sater, Chris Verdery, Willie Cooper, Dr. Al Oppenheim, Dr. Bill Barfield, Jay Sanders, David Rivers, Scott Shearouse.

And several helpful anonymouses. You know who you are. Thank you, everyone. Thank you very much.

ABOUT THE AUTHOR

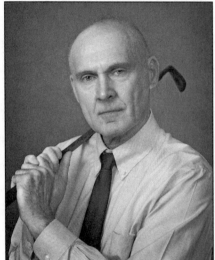

Photo by Bruce Lattimer

Curt Sampson, golf professional turned golf writer, came to golf the old-fashioned way—as a caddie. He looped for his father for a few years on summer Saturdays, then turned pro, in a manner of speaking, at age twelve, as one of the scores of disheveled boys and men in the caddie pen at Lake Forest Country Club in Hudson, Ohio. His golf game developed from sneaking onto the course at LFCC at twilight, an occasionally nerve-wracking exercise because the greenskeeper intimated a readiness to call the cops on trespassers. Sampson—never caught—progressed as a player and as an employee, scoring a job as starter/cart maintenance boy at age 16 at Boston Hills CC—a public course—also in Hudson. His high-water mark as a young golfer was a win in the Mid-American Junior in 1970. Sampson attended Kent State University on a golf scholarship and managed a municipal course for two years following graduation, worked a couple more as an assistant pro at clubs in South Carolina and Tennessee, then bummed around as a touring pro in Canada, New Zealand, and Florida.

In November 1988, Sampson began to write full-time, mostly about the game of his father, golf. *Texas Golf Legends*, his first book, was a collaboration with Santa Fe-based artist Paul Milosevich. Researching that book gained Sampson introductions with people he has written about many times since: Ben Hogan, Byron Nelson, Ben Crenshaw, Lee Trevino, and a few dozen others. His next book, *The Eternal Summer*—a re-creation of golf's summer of 1960, when Hogan, Arnold Palmer, and Jack Nicklaus battled—is still selling 27 years after its debut, a rarity in the publishing world. Sampson's biography of the enigmatic William Ben Hogan struck a chord. Both *Hogan* and his next book, *The Masters*, appeared on the *New York Times* bestseller lists. Subsequent books and scores of magazine articles cemented Sampson's reputation as readable and sometimes controversial writer with an eye for humor and the telling detail. *Roaring Back* is Sampson's eighteenth book.

He lives in the Dallas-Fort Worth area.

INDEX

INDEX

251